The Physicist's Guide to Weight Loss

Buesing, Mark M.

The Physicist's Guide to Weight Loss – 1st Edition

Illustrated by Mark Buesing

ISBN 978-0-6151-4858-8

Dedicated to the memory of my father – Merrill Buesing.

The best parts of me, I owe to him.

Disclaimer

No weight loss or weight gain program should be considered or begun without first consulting your physician or health care professional.

Table of Contents

Preface

A few years ago I was sitting around the Thanksgiving Day table with my father, mother, sister, brother-in-law, and wife. As is often the case during the holidays, the subject turned to weight loss or more accurately weight *gain*. This was the perfect opportunity for one of my rants about how silly all the diet books are. Each book says theirs is the only way to effectively lose weight: high carbohydrate this and low protein that, you have to eat more of these or eat less of those, etc. Each book contradicts the next. How does the average person know whom to believe? I even joked I was going to write a book about losing weight on an all butter diet. I was really poking fun at all the diet books.

I kept saying it was just basic physics. Plain and simple losing or gaining weight is basic conservation of energy, just like you (hopefully) learned in grade school. You know, "Energy can neither be created nor destroyed ..." Distilled down to its most basic elements, weight loss and weight gain are easily understood and mastered. Everyone at the table listened patiently and when I finished my ranting they said in unison, "If *you're* so smart why don't you write a book."

So I did. I hope you like it.

Chapter 1

UNDERSTANDING WEIGHT LOSS AND WEIGHT GAIN

This is the only chapter you really need to read. No kidding. I never understood why weight loss books are so long. Whether you lose or gain weight is governed by the simplest of physical laws, and there's no escaping it. To understand whether you will lose or gain weight requires only the most basic of physics - physics that can be explained in one chapter.

People are often afraid of physics. Maybe they had a bad experience in high school; maybe they think it's all mathematics; or worse yet, maybe they think it doesn't apply to their everyday lives. Nothing could be further from the truth. This book will give you a warm, fuzzy feeling about physics, show you that the mathematics is easy, and most importantly, show you that physics plays a vital role in your everyday life, especially when it comes to weight loss and weight gain.

Judging by the sheer number of weight loss books and the number of different diets, weight loss and weight gain must be a very misunderstood physics principle. It is amazing that one diet says you must limit a certain food group to lose weight and the very next says you must *maximize* the same food group to lose weight. It doesn't have to be that way. The physics of weight loss (and weight gain) is easily understood. There is only one basic physics principle that needs to be understood. There is no magic diet that works and none that is doomed to fail. Each diet works or doesn't work based on one very simple and basic physics principle called the Conservation of Energy.

Certain irrefutable laws govern our universe. Paramount among these is the Conservation of Energy. You probably learned this in sixth grade:

> "Energy can neither be created nor destroyed, only changed from one form to another."

We must also define *energy* in the physics sense. Energy is the ability to do work, so any work done has to come from some available supply of energy. Work is what you think it is. Lifting, walking, and even reading this book are all work. Just as importantly for weight loss, your body also does work all the time. Breathing, pumping blood, and maintaining a temperature of 98.6°F are all work, too. Work in physics is like work in your everyday life. Every time work gets done there must be some energy expenditure.

Now let's apply these simple physics ideas to weight loss and weight gain. Let's say this is you:

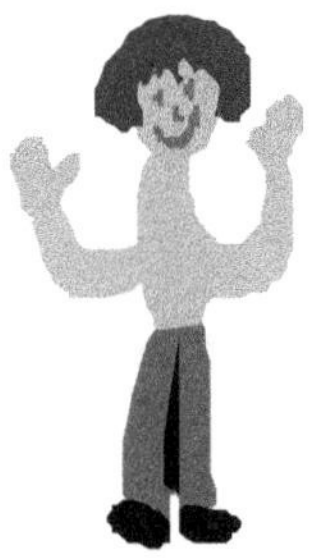

Physicists are famous for simplifying things, so let's simplify the picture of you to this *model* of you:

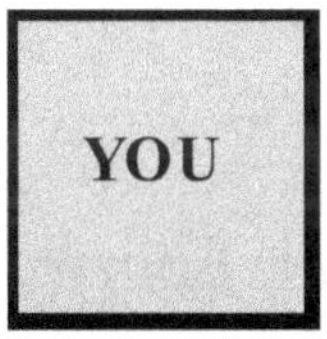

Yes, that's you. Your outer appearance, personality, and even the content of your character don't influence the laws of physics and whether you gain or lose weight. Now let's look at how the human body deals with energy.

The energy required to do everything the human body does comes from the food you eat and drink. There is only one way for energy to get in to your body, and that's through the food you put in your mouth. Energy is not absorbed through the skin or created inside the body. It comes in through your mouth in the form of chemical potential energy in the food you eat. That's it. Period. There is no deeper understanding or magic formulas. Let me just say that again so you see how simple this idea of weight loss/gain really is: **The energy your body uses comes only from the food you put in your mouth**.

So let's add one element to our model of you:

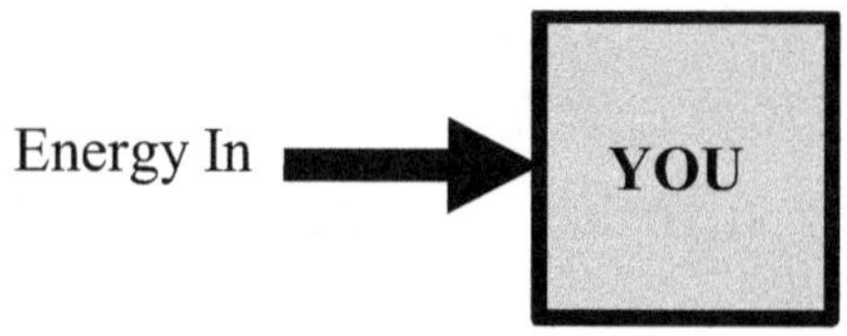

Now that wouldn't be the complete picture because if you only put things in, you would gain weight your whole life. So, we need to add one more element to our model of you, Energy Out:

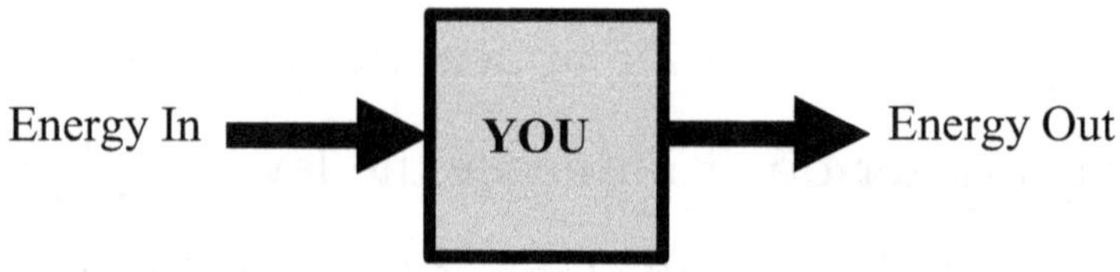

Physics and the conservation of energy are easy to understand. If the Energy In is greater than the Energy Out, then you will gain weight. If the Energy In is less than the Energy Out, then you will lose weight. If the Energy In equals the Energy Out, then you maintain your weight. That's it.

This simple relationship is called the Conservation of Energy, and it cannot be violated. In summary:

Energy In	greater than	Energy Out	Weight Gain
Energy In	less than	Energy Out	Weight Loss
Energy In	equal to	Energy Out	Maintain Weight

Think of it like these seesaws:

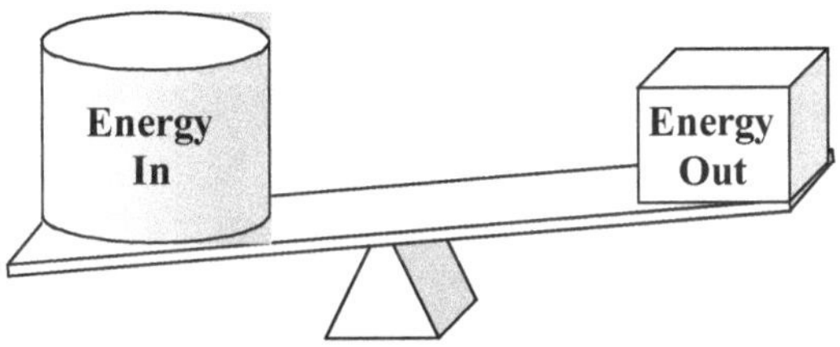

Weight Gain

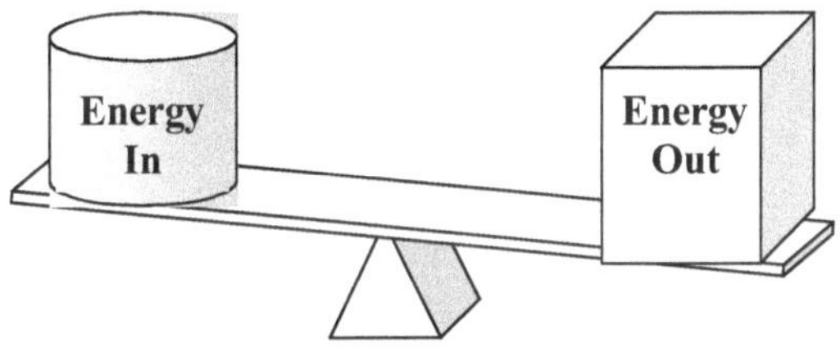

Weight Loss

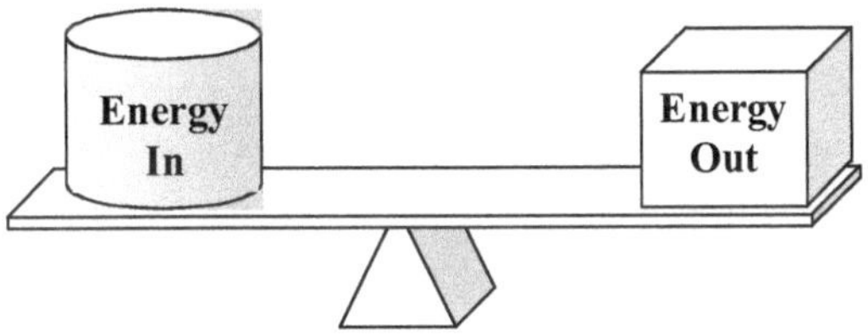

Maintain Weight

This is the only physics you have to understand to determine whether you will gain or lose weight. It doesn't matter what diet you follow or how active you are. If you take in more energy than you expend, you will gain weight. If you expend more energy than you take in, you lose weight. If you take in what you expend, then your weight doesn't change.

That's it for the physics. The Conservation of Energy rules our universe and your body. It's simple. You have the basics; now it's time to get a little more specific.

Chapter 2

BMR AND WORK

Energy is used by your body for two things. First, energy is used by your body for basic functioning, everything from breathing, to making your heart beat, to cell reproduction, and a large part is used just maintaining a body temperature of 98.6°F. The sum total of all this energy expenditure is called your Basal Metabolic Rate, or BMR. It's how many Calories your body needs per day just to maintain its proper functioning.

It's a fairly easy number to calculate (we'll do that in a minute). The second thing energy is used for is all the work you do in your daily activities like driving, walking, standing, swimming, typing, holding this book, running, lifting weights, aerobics class, climbing stairs, etc. That's it – two things.

To summarize: The energy you put into your body in the form of food you eat (Energy In) is used to keep your body functioning (BMR) and also used to do exercise (Work). Our simple picture of you now looks like this:

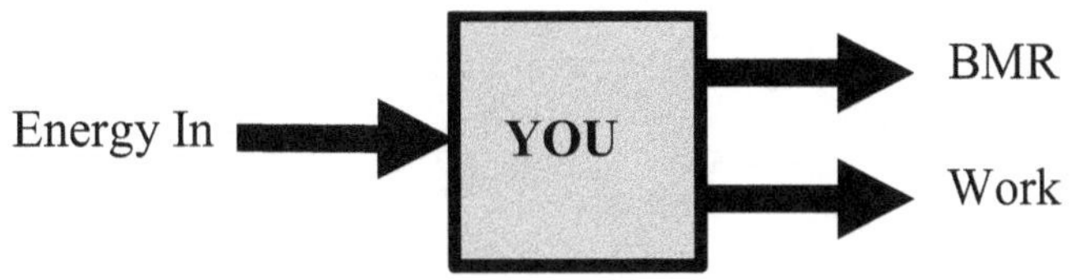

The Conservation of Energy still applies. If the Energy In is greater than the total of the Basal Metabolic Rate plus Work then, you will gain weight. If the Energy In is less than the total of the Basal Metabolic Rate plus Work, then you will lose weight. If the Energy In equals the total of the Basal Metabolic Rate plus Work, then you maintain your weight. That's it. And I promise it doesn't get any more complicated. To summarize:

Energy In	**greater than**	**BMR + Work**	**Weight Gain**
Energy In	**less than**	**BMR + Work**	**Wright Loss**
Energy In	**equal to**	**BMR + Work**	**Maintain Weight**

Or, look at it like a seesaw again:

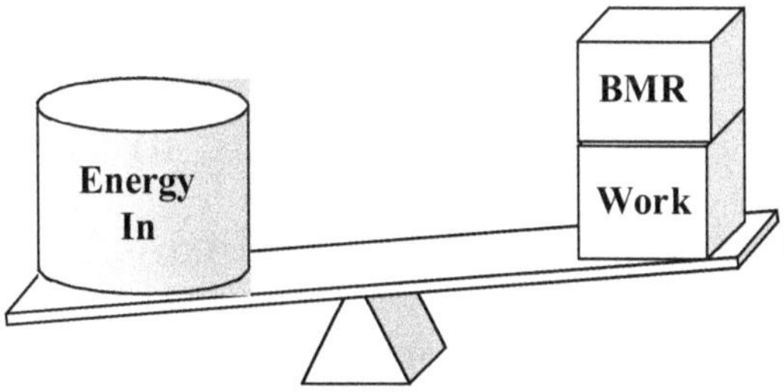

Weight Gain

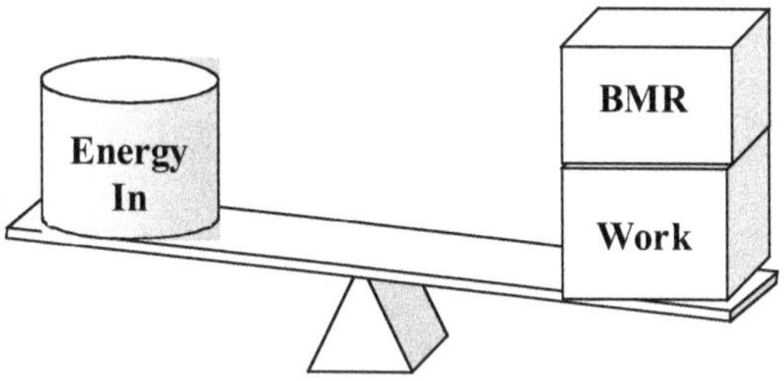

Weight Loss

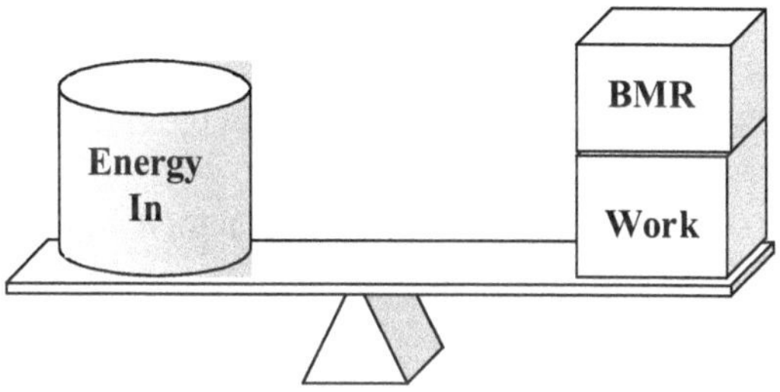

Maintain Weight

Now that you have the basic physics, we are going to look more closely at the three factors that determine whether you gain or lose weight: Energy In, Basal Metabolic Rate, and Work.

First, Energy In. Energy only comes into your body one way: through the food you put in your mouth. That's it. Energy is not absorbed through your skin or somehow created inside your body. Sure, it's transformed inside your body from one form to another, but the only way your body gets energy is by putting food in your mouth; there's no other way.

How do you determine how much energy you are putting in your body? You can either use the Calorie tables in **Appendix B – Calories/kcal Tables** or read the food labels on the products you eat and drink and total up how much energy measured in Calories you are putting in your body every day. Yep, it's that simple. Energy only comes in through your mouth, so all you have to do is keep track of the total.

Second, your Basal Metabolic Rate. You'll need a calculator (I promise the math is easy), your current weight in pounds, your height in inches, and your age (don't lie!). Then, perform one of the following calculations:

Men:

$$BMR = 66 + (6.23 \times \text{weight}) + (12.7 \times \text{height}) - (6.8 \times \text{age})$$

Women:

$$BMR = 655 + (4.36 \times \text{weight}) + (4.57 \times \text{height}) - (4.7 \times \text{age})$$

If your math is a little rusty let's do a quick example. You are a woman who weighs 175 pounds, is 5 feet 4 inches tall, and is 40 years old. First, convert your height to inches by multiplying 5 times 12 and adding 4, resulting in 64 inches. Substitute your weight, height, and age into the formula and compute:

$$BMR = 665 + (4.36 \times 175) + (4.57 \times 64) - (4.7 \times 40)$$
$$BMR = 665 + (763) + (292) - (188)$$
$$BMR = 1532$$

Now repeat the calculation using your own weight, height, and age. Write this number down; you'll need it later.

This is *your* Basal Metabolic Rate measured in Calories. It gives you a rough idea of how many Calories you use every day just to maintain your body's proper functioning. True, two people who are the same weight, height, and age may have different basal metabolic rates, but this number gives us a starting point. What does it mean? In our example, even if you stay in bed all day and you eat fewer than 1532 Calories you will lose weight. Do some work or exercise and you lose even more!

Finally, your body uses energy to do work. Walking, standing, typing, exercising, and even holding this book require energy. To figure out how much energy a particular activity uses, just look it up in **Appendix A - Work Out / METs Tables**. The appendix lists all sorts of activities. You just have to total up all your daily expenditures. Most electronic exercise equipment like treadmills, elliptical trainers, stair climbers, and stationary bikes will display how many Calories you expended as long as you input your weight in the beginning. Using the Calories from the exercise equipment is probably more accurate than using Appendix A.

No kidding - that's it. Three things alone determine if you gain or lose weight. The Basal Metabolic Rate calculation is performed only once, so on a daily basis you only have to keep track of Energy In (food Calories) and Work (exercise).

Remember, if you are trying to lose weight, then it's always better to slightly over-estimate your Energy In (food Calories) and underestimate your Work (exercise duration and intensity). There's not much you can do about your Basal Metabolic Rate, so losing or gaining weight becomes a simple game of balancing Energy In with Work.

What your grandmother told you is true: weight loss is a matter of diet and exercise. There's just no way around the Conservation of Energy.

Chapter 3

HOW MUCH WILL I LOSE?

How do you determine how much weight you'll lose or gain? Each pound of body fat contains 3500 Calories of energy. That means that each pound of body fat can do 3500 Calories of Work. In other words, you need to output 3500 Calories more than you input to lose one pound of body fat. A deficit of 3500 Calories to lose *one* pound of body weight? I know it seems like a lot, but there's no escaping the laws of physics. That energy (body fat) didn't just appear. It was input one bite at a time, and it is going to take some work (literally) to get rid of it.

Let's make it a little easier on you. On the next pages are a simple worksheet you can use followed by an example worksheet. Make some copies of the blank one so you can keep track of weight gain or loss on a daily basis.

Breakfast:

Food	Calories	Food	Calories

Lunch:

Food	Calories	Food	Calories

Dinner:

Food	Calories	Food	Calories

Snacks:

Food	Calories

Total Energy In (Food Calories)	+	

BMR	-	

Work:

Activity	Calories

Total Work	-	
Daily Total (Total of Above)	±	

Daily Total ÷ 3500 = Pounds Lost (-) or Gained (+)	±	
Total to Date	±	

Breakfast:

Food	Calories	Food	Calories
cereal - 2 cups	**200**		
skim milk - 1 cup	**90**		
orange juice - 1 cup	**110**		

Lunch:

Food	Calories	Food	Calories
turkey sand on wheat		**granola bar**	**110**
w/ lettuce & tomato	**300**	**diet cola**	**0**
tortilla chips - 1 cup	**140**		

Dinner:

Food	Calories	Food	Calories
chicken breast no skin	**160**	**skim milk - 1 cup**	**90**
spaghetti - 3 oz.	**300**	**peas/carrots-1/2 cup**	**50**
spag. sauce - 1/2 cup	**140**		

Snacks:

Food	Calories
candy bar	**210**
apple - medium	**80**

Total Energy In (Food Calories)	+	**1980**

BMR	-	**1532**

Work:

Activity	Calories
walking - 30 min	**183**
elliptical trainer - 30 min	**359**
grocery shopping - 30 min	**100**

Total Work	-	**642**
Daily Total (Total of Above)	-	**194**

Daily Total ÷ 3500 = Pounds Lost (-) or Gained (+)	-	**0.055**
Total to Date	±	

Simply write down all the foods you eat during the day and total them in the Total Energy In (Food Calories) box. This is a positive number because it is Energy *In*. In the BMR box put your Basal Metabolic Rate you calculated in Chapter 2. This is a negative number because it's Energy *Out*. Next, total all your work in the form of daily activities and exercise and write it in for Total Work. This is another negative number. From Total Energy In (Food Calorie) subtract BMR and subtract Total Work. Write this number in the Daily Total (Total of Above). The Daily Total tells you how many Calories you are over (if it's positive), or how many Calories you are under (if it's negative). Divide Daily Total by 3500, and you have the actual weight loss or weight gain for that day.

What? Only 0.055 pounds lost! Yes, but do the math: -0.055 multiplied by 30 days is -1.65 pounds. 1.65 multiplied by 12 months in a year equals **20** pounds lost. That's a lot! Not good enough for you? Want to lose more? Skip the candy bar and you lose 0.12 pounds per day, 3.6 pounds per month, and **43** pounds in a year! Either way, that's amazing. You could be a whole new person inside of a year. Our 175 pound example is somewhere between 155 and 132 pounds one year from now.

Don't kid yourself; it's going to be tough. It's not going to be easy snacking on just one apple every day. And be careful; skip the 30 minutes on the elliptical *and* eat the candy bar, you now have an *excess* of 165 Calories, +0.047 pounds per day, +1.41 pounds in a month, and +16.5 pounds in a year. Our 175 pound example now weighs 191.5 pounds.

Make no mistake: It's going to take a change of lifestyle to accomplish significant weight loss. You have to tip that seesaw in your favor every day. It's the little things that add up.

Every day you lose weight is a day you didn't gain weight.

Chapter 4

HOW MUCH SHOULD I LOSE?

How much weight should you lose? Your body mass index (BMI) is an easy way of determining how much you should lose to lead a healthy life. It's another calculation, but it's simple. You'll need your height in inches and weight in pounds again. To calculate your BMI perform the following calculation (it's the same for men and women):

$$BMI = \frac{705 \times weight}{(height \times height)}$$

Let's do another example. Once again, imagine you are 5 feet 4 inches tall (64 inches) and weigh 175 pounds.

$$BMI = \frac{705 \times 175}{(64 \times 64)}$$

$$BMI = \frac{705 \times 175}{4096}$$

$$BMI = 30.1$$

Now use the chart to determine which category you fit into:

BMI	description	risk of disease
less than 20	underweight	
20-25	normal	low
25-30	overweight	moderate
greater than 30	obese	high

The BMI calculations are used by insurance companies and medical professionals to determine ideal weight and asses your risk of certain diseases associated with excess weight like heart disease, certain cancers, diabetes, etc.

Working backwards, we can determine a goal weight for our example:

$$\text{goal weight} = \frac{25 \times (\text{height} \times \text{height})}{705}$$

$$\text{goal weight} = \frac{25 \times (64 \times 64)}{705}$$

$$\text{goal weight} = \frac{25 \times 4096}{705}$$

$$\text{goal weight} = 145$$

To determine your own goal weight just plug *your* height into the sample calculation above. This gives you the upper limit of the normal weight range. To calculate the lower limit of the normal range, change the 25 to a 20 and recompute with your height.

Don't weigh yourself every day. Your body weight fluctuates significantly from hydration and whether you have recently used the bathroom. Instead, weigh yourself once a week in the morning (you are usually a bit dehydrated in the morning) after using the bathroom (more realistic body weight) and without clothes on (why add another variable to the equation). You should see a close agreement with what your weekly total is from the worksheets. If not, there could be several reasons:

- Make sure you are keeping track of *everything* that goes in your mouth. Be realistic about serving sizes. No one eats 3/4 cup of cereal for breakfast like the box says—it's probably 2 cups or more! Measure your portions with a measuring cup to check.

- Be conservative about your energy output. Are you getting off the treadmill to change the channel? Pausing drops your heart rate. Are you really walking 20-minute miles? Be realistic.

- You might need to add a "fudge factor" to your basal metabolic rate—but don't do this until you have a month worth of data and you've been careful about keeping track of Energy In and Work Out. If you are being accurate with everything and still gaining weight (or not losing as much as you should), then multiply your basal metabolic rate by 0.9. If, after another month your numbers still aren't agreeing, then multiply by 0.8.

- As you lose weight (and gain age) you will have to recalculate your basal metabolic rate periodically.

- If you are actually losing more than you are predicting, then multiply your basal metabolism by 1.1 and see if that helps bring your prediction in alignment with what you are seeing on the scale every week, or leave it alone because you are heading in the right direction!

What, no talk about carbohydrates, fats, or proteins? No. No matter what diet you follow, they must all follow the Conservation of Energy. It doesn't matter what mix of foods you eat; it's all about balancing the Energy In (food Calories) with the Energy Out (BMR and Work). Follow whatever diet you want: low carb, low fat, low glycemic index; it doesn't matter. In order to lose weight on any diet you must follow the Conservation of Energy. You could eat an all-butter diet (I don't recommend it!) and lose weight as long as your Caloric intake was less than your Caloric output.

What do I recommend? I'm just a physicist, so consult your doctor. Always discuss any weight loss program with a medical professional before you begin. Ask your doctor if you have any specific dietary restrictions or health issues that will affect you. After that, do what your grandmother told you. Eat a lot of fruits and veggies (not a lot of calories but a lot of good nutrients); eat and drink all things in moderation; limit the sugar and fat; and follow the United States Department of Agriculture's food pyramid:

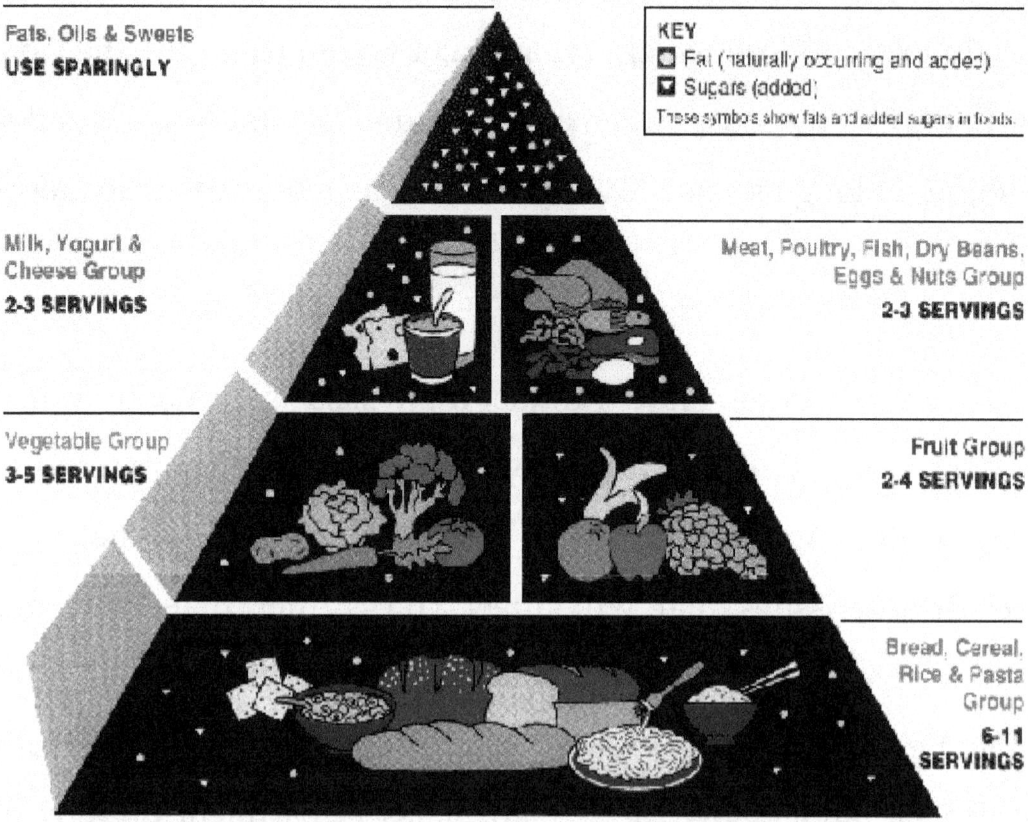

Your federal government has spent millions of your tax dollars studying nutrition. Some of the best scientists in the world have worked at USDA labs across the country. These people know nutrition and what your body needs to maintain a healthy life. Use some common sense. Trust the Conservation of Energy and what your grandmother told you. Eat right and exercise—it's really that simple.

In 2005 the United States Department of Agriculture came out with a new pyramid that is much more individualized. The new pyramid can be found at http://www.mypyramid.gov. Input your age, gender, and exercise level, and the web site gives you suggested servings for the various food groups. Definitely check it out. It's free and easy.

So, that's really the end of this book. Compare Energy In (the food you put in your mouth) with your Basal Metabolic Rate and Work (exercise) and you either have weight gain, weight loss, or a balance. It's the Conservation of Energy! It's physics! It's simply how the universe works, and that includes your body.

Okay, I lied. There are other chapters. The next one is on weight loss strategies, the one after that is on motivation, and the other ones are about physics. Besides helping people understand their own bodies and weight gain and weight loss, I've always wanted to help people understand physics. It's an amazing subject and it's *easy*. Read on - you'll burn a couple Calories in the process!

Chapter 5

WEIGHT LOSS STRATEGIES

Losing some weight is accomplished by most of the people who start a diet. Keeping the weight off is accomplished by only about 5% of the people who start a diet. You have a better chance of getting hooked on heroin and quitting than maintaining your weight loss. That's because weight loss is a *permanent lifestyle change*. You can't follow your plan for a few months, lose some weight, and then go back to your old habits, because you'll gain weight again.

There are only three things that happen every day: weight loss, no change, or weight gain. It's the Conservation of Energy. It's that simple. In order to maintain your weight loss you have to *permanently* change your habits. You have to understand the Conservation of Energy and understand there's no escaping the simple physics of it. That seesaw is going to tip one way or the other!

This chapter lists some strategies to help you lose weight. Most are very sensible, and a couple are a bit off-the-wall.

- Set specific goals. It's not going to work if your goal is "to lose some weight" or "get in shape." Your goals need to be very specific. "I want to lose 32 pounds" or "I am going to walk 4 miles every day but Tuesday" or "I am going to eat only one cookie per day" are specific goals. The more specific in time, space, and weight you can be, the better.

- To increase your metabolic rate you can get younger (not likely), get taller (see getting younger), or gain weight. Gain weight! That's what you are trying to avoid. Seriously, if you can gain lean body mass, i.e., muscle, you can increase your basal metabolic rate. Pump some iron!

  Put together a strength training program and make it a habit. Strength training really helps tip the seesaw to the weight loss side. It affects both your BMR and Work. Think about it. You are lifting weights (Work) so you are expending Calories *and* you are helping to build lean body mass (muscle), which will increase your BMR. Don't worry about gaining more muscle weight than you lose in body fat. If the right side of the seesaw (BMR and Work) is greater than the left side (Energy In) you will still lose weight no matter how much you lift. If you build muscle and lose weight at the same time you can really accelerate the rate at which you will drop those excess pounds.

- You don't need a fancy gym or fancy equipment to put together a strength program. Sure, if you have the disposable income and time, join a gym. You can even hire a personal trainer, but you don't *need* to. You can buy weight sets at garage sales or make your own out of milk jugs filled with water or sand. Heismann Trophy winner Herschel Walker decided he'd get into shape by doing push-ups, sit-ups, squats, etc. during commercial breaks while he watched television one summer. He didn't lift a single weight other than his own body weight. At the end of one summer of doing this he made his high school football team, and the rest is collegiate and NFL history.

- Get someone to start a lifestyle change, I mean "weight loss program", with you. Being part of a group, even if it's only a pair, is going to increase your chance of making your changes permanent. You are much more likely to get out the door at 5:30 a.m. for a three mile walk if you know your neighbor is waiting for you. My dad always said company loves misery!

- Read food labels. Read food labels. Read food labels. Spend some time in the grocery store reading the labels on the products you buy. You only have to look at two things: Calories and serving size. By law every product sold has to contain this basic information. Serving size and Calories are shown below on a standard label:

Nutrition Facts

Serving Size 17 Crackers (30g)
Servings Per Container About 15

Amount Per Serving	
Calories 140	Calories from Fat 50
	% Daily Value*
Total Fat 6g	**9%**
Saturated Fat 2.5g	**13%**
Trans Fat 0g	
Cholesterol 0mg	**0%**
Sodium 270mg	**11%**
Total Carbohydrate 19g	**6%**
Dietary Fiber less than 1g	**1%**
Sugars 0g	
Protein 2g	

Vitamin A 4%	Vitamin C 0%
Calcium 0%	Iron 8%

* Percent Daily Values are based on a 2,000 calorie diet. Your daily values may be higher or lower depending on your calorie needs:

	Calories	2,000	2,500
Total Fat	Less than	65g	80g
Sat. Fat	Less than	20g	25g
Cholesterol	Less than	300mg	300mg
Sodium	Less than	2,400mg	2,400mg
Total Carbohydrate		300g	375g
Dietary Fiber		25g	30g

- You have to look at Calories, because that's what you are going to write in your table. You have to look at serving size, because you want to compare products on an even playing field. If you are looking to buy granola bars, find the one that gives you the least Calories for an equal serving size. It gets a little tricky, because not all serving sizes are equal. 28 grams (or 1 ounce) is a fairly standard serving size, but is not universal. Some manufacturers try to make their products appear more appealing by shrinking the serving size. Look through the candy bar isle.

You'll find a couple that list their candy bar as *two* servings. Yeah, right, like I'm only going to eat half the candy bar once I unwrap it!

Sure, you might have to take your calculator to the grocery store, but that's okay — people will think you are a physicist writing a book about weight loss!

You mean there's no talk about carbs, fats, or proteins? Nope. Calories are the only thing that determines weight loss or gain. All the high this and low that diets work only if they follow the conservation of energy. If your BMR and Work are greater than Energy In, then any specific diet will work.

- Be truthful about serving size. If the package says there are 10 servings and you finish it in 5 sittings, then you are eating 2 servings at a time. Get it? I eat cereal most mornings. The box says there are 12 servings at 110 Calories per serving. I use a big bowl for cereal, and I finish the box in four days. That means I am actually eating *triple* servings (12÷4=3). On my worksheet I have to write down 330 Calories (110x3=330) for cereal. It's like this with a lot of products. Some microwave popcorns list 3 servings per bag. If you eat the whole bag yourself (who doesn't?) then you have to triple the Calories.

- Park in the back of the lot at work or the mall. If it takes you an extra couple minutes of walking, you are tipping that seesaw. Avoid elevators and escalators. Climbing stairs is a great workout. And, of course, *never* take the moving sidewalk at the airport!

- Put your power tools away and work like your grandfather. Dust off your handsaw and go to work. Put away the cordless driver and use your screwdrivers again.

- Look for ways to do more physical work. Wash your car by hand. Get off the riding mower. I know it takes more time, but you have to find some activities that you can make a *habit*. Be creative and find some things you enjoy that require physical labor. Get some calluses and break a few nails!

- Want to try a crazy idea? Sleep with fewer covers. If you use two blankets, take one off. If you only have one, use only the sheet or a thinner blanket. You are in for a miserable week or two because you are going to be cold at night. Resist the urge to cover up, because if you can stick it out for a week or so your body will begin to adjust by increasing its Basal Metabolic Rate at night to keep you warm. Yep, you'll burn more Calories, even while you sleep! You'll also amaze yourself by being able to sleep comfortably with next to nothing over you.

- Exercise in the cold. Your body not only has to do the normal work of exercise, but also work a bit harder keeping your body at 98.6°F. Studies have shown that you use about 10% more Calories when it's cold outside than when it's warm. Of course ,use some common sense – don't risk injury or frostbite to burn a couple more Calories.

- Don't ever try to "sweat pounds off." Any water lost through perspiration and evaporation is not actually "lost." Weight can only be lost on that seesaw. Work and BMR have to be greater than food Calories In. Dehydrating yourself is not only temporary (the weight comes back as soon as you rehydrate your body) – it's dangerous. Becoming dehydrated not only makes you feel awful, it decreases your ability to continue exercising, and in the worst case can kill you. Drink plenty of fluids before, during, and after exercise and remember: It's Conservation of Energy, not dehydration, that leads to weight loss.

- All these ideas can help, but remember—it has to be a *permanent* lifestyle change. If you only stick to your plan for a few months or even a few years, it will work during that time. If you slip back into your old habits, you will eventually wind up back where you started.

Chapter 6

NEED SOME MOTIVATION?

Make the decision today that you are going to lose weight, and that's it. Decision done. Once you've made the decision to lose weight then it is a personal commitment governed by your character. Do you have the character to follow through? Do you have the character to stick with it when it's difficult? When it's really, really difficult? You do. Don't disappoint yourself. It's not a good feeling when you disappoint yourself, and you're stronger that that.

You can do it. Keep it simple. Limit the Energy In and maximize the Work Out. Tip that seesaw to the Work Out side and you are going to lose weight. Imagine yourself losing weight. See yourself shedding body mass one-hundredth of a pound at a time. It came in one forkful at a time, so it's going to have to come off the same way. Tiny steps add up. You have to have patience.

I hear people say weight gain is so easy and weight loss is so hard. It just isn't so. It only seems hard because the human attention span is so short. People want it now or forget it. You have to be better than that. You have to have faith in yourself; you have to have the strength of character to get through the tough times; and you have to understand the Conservation of Energy.

Let's say you've gained 60 pounds since high school, and that was 20 years ago. That means you've gained an average of 0.008 pounds per day. That means you ate, on average, +28 extra Calories per day for 20 years. Did it seem easy? Sure, because it seems like those pounds just showed up all of a sudden. That just isn't so. Those 60 pounds came in one mouthful at a time, +28 Calories extra per day, to be exact. To make losing weight as easy as gaining weight you should take those pounds off 0.008 per day for 20 years.

I know, that's not realistic. No one has *that* kind of patience. What's realistic? It depends on you and your doctor. Sixty pounds in one year means .16 pounds per day or -560 Calories. That's pretty ambitious and could be dangerous. Sixty pounds in 2 years is 0.08 pounds per day or -280 Calories per day. But 2 years is a long time, you say! Let's not kid ourselves – it might take 2 years to lose 60 pounds. You have to believe in yourself. You have to have the strength of character to be disciplined. You have to have patience. You have to make *permanent* changes.

You can't get around the Conservation of Energy; you have to work with it. Weight loss can be accomplished only by making your BMR and Work greater than your Energy In. You can do it if you understand that every day you tip the seesaw in your favor is one step toward your goal. Keep stepping!

Losing weight is not easy. Since our universe is governed by the Conservation of Energy that means gaining weight is equally hard. You have to run or walk 35 miles to expend the 3500 Calories it takes to lose one pound of body mass. But it also took 7 large, double hamburgers with cheese and extra sauce to gain that same 3500 Calories or one pound of body mass. Metabolism doesn't matter; you still had to go over your Caloric needs by 3500 Calories.

So how do you stay motivated to keep making good food choices? Remember that every pound you want to lose came in through your mouth. The fewer Calories you put in, the fewer you have to worry about working out. Look back at the simplified model of your body. Energy In goes to BMR and Work. That's it. Don't make it more complicated. Keep it simple. You can't do much for metabolism except lift weights to gain some muscle. This will help you a little (and every Calorie counts), but it's Energy In (food Calories) and Work (exercise) that matter the most. When you reach for that candy bar, equate that to your preferred exercise and figure out how many minutes (or hours) you'll be at it. If you have a family, job, social life, hobby, or just like sitting around—think twice!

Use visualization. Use those hunger feelings as your cue. Wait … did I just say hunger feelings? You bet, and some people even call them hunger *pains.* Your body has a built-in defense mechanism. It knows that you can't tip the seesaw forever. If your BMR and Work were greater than Energy In long enough, you would eventually starve to death. Your body knows this, and it certainly doesn't want to die, so it sends signals to eat more. Ignore those signals! No, it's not easy, but use those signals to start visualizing yourself losing weight. See yourself shedding pounds. Imagine yourself getting lighter, getting thinner, and more importantly—healthier. Every time you feel hungry, congratulate yourself. You're doing it. Also, take refuge in the fact that those feelings will be most acute in the beginning. As time goes on those feelings will subside. It might take a couple weeks, but they will definitely be a lot less in no time.

Reward yourself along the way, but don't use food as your reward. If you are trying to break old habits and form new habits, using food as your incentive is not doing yourself any favors. I have never fed my dog human food, and the not so amazing thing is that he's not interested in human food at all. I have friends say that I'm mean because I don't give him a human food treat once in a while. I argue the exact opposite. I say it is meaner to "tease" him with human food. Since I never feed my dog human food, then he is happy with dog food and doesn't even know there is another kind of food. Make it the same way with your new habits. Either cut a food out entirely or incorporate it reasonably into a new habit, but don't tease yourself with food.

Make your rewards something personal: A new pair of jeans, time alone, a tanning session, a gym membership, a vacation to show off your new body. Make it something that will make you feel better about yourself. It doesn't have to cost money. Send the kids to the neighbors, take a bubble bath, and watch something mindless on television. Incorporate specific rewards into your specific goals. "When I have gone 20 straight days in the negative, I am going to treat myself to an afternoon walk in the park by myself." If that's hokey, then come up with your own!

Imagine yourself at your goal weight. Visualize what you will look like. Visualize how you will feel. Now divide the distance from now to then by many steps and visualize yourself on that path. Every day you will be looking and feeling better. Sure you only look and feel 0.08 pounds better every day, but there are 365.24 days in a year, and that means 26 pounds in a year!

Once you get to your goal weight then you have an additional reward. You no longer need to tip the seesaw. Now you *balance* it! I highly encourage you not to decrease the Work, but slightly increase the Energy In. Be careful and do the math. It might only mean you get an extra banana per day. You will never be able to go back to your old ways. It's got to be a *permanent* lifestyle change. You can do it! Have patience, believe in yourself, and tell yourself you have the strength of character to permanently change. The journey of a thousand miles begins with a single step – so get stepping (literally)!

The next few chapters deal with physics. Physics is what I live, breath, and teach everyday. I love it. By reading the next few chapters you will learn more about the world in which you live. You can also skip over these chapters (for now) and go right to the Calorie / kcal Tables in Appendix A; I won't be too offended.

Chapter 7

MASS VS. WEIGHT

These two words are the most mixed up words in the English language. They are not the same things although most people think they are. To a physicist they mean two different things.

Mass is the amount of matter in an object. Literally the total amount of protons, neutrons, and electrons in an object. Mass is the quantitative measure of the inertia of an object. Inertia is how hard it is to get an object to move; or conversely, once it's moving how hard it is to get it to stop. (Don't mix this up with momentum—momentum is an object's mass multiplied by its velocity.) The mass of an object never changes unless you remove part of it or add to it. It's a fundamental quantity.

Weight, on the other hand, is a force due to gravity. A force is a push or pull. The weight of an object depends on where it is in relation to other things with mass. The weight of an object is calculated from other quantities. The formula is $F_g = mg$ where F_g is weight, m is mass and g is the acceleration due to gravity. You need to redo the calculation if you move the object to a different location in the universe (or strictly speaking, even to the top of a tall building).

Let's say the mass of an object is 70 kilograms, the mass of the average person. No matter where you go in the universe your mass will still be 70 kg. Even if you go to a microgravity (near zero g) environment, your mass is still 70 kg. It takes just as much force to get you moving or to stop you once you are moving in deep space as it does on earth. However, your weight will change depending on where you are. On earth your 70 kg mass weighs about 700 Newtons (the Newton is the unit of weight in the metric system), on Jupiter you weigh 1,800 N, on the moon you weigh 120 Newtons, and in a microgravity environment you are weightless (0 N).

Interestingly enough, the shuttle astronauts are not weightless because of a lack of gravity in orbit. There's about 93% of the gravity at space shuttle altitudes as there is right here on the surface of the earth. They are weightless because they are literally free falling like you would be in an elevator if the cables were cut! The shuttle doesn't fall into the earth because it has a very large tangential speed (speed around the earth). So we say the shuttle falls *around* the earth and the astronauts are weightless because they are falling! Imagine being on a ride like the Giant Drop at Six Flags for a couple weeks, 24 hours a day and 7 days per week!

Why go into this explanation? Because strictly speaking, you want to lose mass. You can reduce your weight simply by going to the top of a tall building. At the top of the Sears Tower in Chicago you'll weigh about one fiftieth of a pound less! (You could lose a bit more by walking to the top!) If you go to the moon you would weigh a lot less—only one-sixth as much as you do on earth. Don't go to Jupiter, though; you'll weigh 2.6 times more than you do on earth.

So losing *weight* is not what you want to do. You actually want to lose *mass*. You want less matter making you up. The title of this book should really be called *The Physicist's Guide to Mass Loss*.

<u>Chapter 8</u>

BATHROOM SCALES, NORMAL FORCES, AND APPARENT WEIGHT

Strictly speaking, bathroom scales don't tell you your weight. They tell you how hard the scale is pushing up against the bottom of your feet. Physicists call this a normal force. It's not normal because other forces are abnormal; normal is another word for perpendicular. Since the scale or any surface can only push perpendicular to itself, physicists say this is a normal force.

There's one more synonym for normal force: *apparent* weight. A bathroom scale measures your apparent weight. You can prove to yourself that bathroom scales don't read your actual weight by standing on a scale while riding up and down in an elevator. When the elevator accelerates upward the scale reading will increase. This is because the scale must push harder against your feet to get you to accelerate upward, too. When the elevator accelerates downward the scale reading will decrease. This is because the scale doesn't have to push as hard against your feet. The scale only reads your true weight when the elevator is not accelerating. When is an elevator not accelerating? When it's not moving, but also when it's moving at a constant velocity.

Next time you buy a bathroom scale, ask the salesperson if the scale reads your weight. When the salesperson answers yes, explain that, no, they really only measure your *apparent* weight. Laugh maniacally as you walk away. Yeah, good fun. Exit the store quickly before store security apprehends you.

Chapter 9

UNITS OF ENERGY

There are three units that physicists typically use when dealing with work, heat, and energy. The standard unit is the Joule (rhymes with "cool"). A Joule is the amount of energy required to lift one kilogram one meter. It's a fairly small unit but the Joule is based on other standard units like the meter and kilogram, so most physicists use it most of the time.

The calorie is a slightly larger unit. It takes 4.2 Joules to make one calorie. The calorie is a convenient unit when working with heat because it takes one calorie of heat energy to raise the temperature of one gram of water one degree centigrade.

The calorie is still a small unit of energy, so sometimes it's easier to work in kilocalories or thousands of calories. To really confuse the issue a kilocalorie or kcal is also known as the Calorie. That's not a misprint; to a physicist there is a difference between calorie and Calorie! Food contains a tremendous amount of chemical potential energy, so when dealing with food it's convenient to use the kcal or Calorie.

In summary, there are 4.2 Joules per calorie and 1000 calories per kcal or 1000 calories per Calorie. One could also say there are 4200 Joules per kcal or Calorie. Simple, huh?

If you really want to make your head spin, the utility companies use the energy unit kilowatt-hours. There are 3,600,000 Joules per kilowatt-hour. That's only 857 Calories per kilowatt-hour though. In most places a kW-hr costs about 10 cents. To light a 100 Watt light bulb for 10 hours takes the equivalent energy of about 3 candy bars.

Chapter 10

WORK

Work is calculated by force multiplied by the distance through which the force acts. The standard unit for work is the Joule. When lifting things the force you use in the calculations is the force due to gravity. Force due to gravity is mass x acceleration due to gravity. Acceleration due to gravity is just a number. 9.8 m/s/s to be exact (on earth). Therefore, if you lift 10 kilograms 1 meter you have done (10)(9.8)(1) or 98 Joules of work.

Using what you learned in Chapter 9, convert Joules to calories by dividing by 4.2 and then convert calories to Calories (kilocalories) by dividing by 1000 and viola—you've just used 0.025 Calories. And a small breath mint is 1 whole Calorie! Whew! Only 40 more lifts to go to burn off that breath mint!

Want a more realistic example? Step up one stair. If your mass is 70 kilograms and the average step is about 20 cm, you just did (70)(9.8)(.20) = 137 Joules of work. To lose one pound of body mass you only need to walk up 107,300 steps. Sure, that's a lot of steps. If this number discourages you remember that you didn't wind up where you are over night. Energy came into your body one mouthful at a time. Remember that next time you reach for a candy bar. If you need help with motivation and starting that journey of 107,300 steps; don't skip Chapter 6!

Seriously, you can now calculate how many Calories you are expending doing exercises not listed in Appendix A. Just follow this formula:

$$\text{Work} = (\text{mass in kilograms})(9.8)(\text{distance in meters})$$

Good calculating!

Chapter 11

Energy and Mass

Energy and mass are two sides of the same coin. It was Albert Einstein who first made this connection in his famous equation $E = mc^2$. Written out, it's Energy equals mass multiplied by the speed of light squared.

The speed of light is 186,000 miles per second, or 300,000,000 meters per second. That's the length of 3,000,000 football fields in one second. While this is the most famous of all physics equations, it is perhaps the most misunderstood. Einstein was not just saying that you can convert mass into energy, he was saying that mass *is* energy. That's an equal sign in the equation. Energy is mass and mass is energy. The speed of light squared is a huge number—almost 100 million trillion. That means there is a tremendous amount of energy in very small amounts of matter. You could supply the energy needs of Los Angeles County for a year from a few kilograms of water.

What does this have to do with weight, I mean, *mass* loss? When you use Calories, your body literally burns some of the stored mass. (Chemists will tell you there was an oxidation reaction.) But it's not what you think. When you run 35 miles you don't lose a pound of fat because you used a pound of fat in your muscles. Your muscles did 3500 Calories or 14,630,000 Joules of work.

Substituting 14,630,000 into $E = mc^2$ looks like this:

$$14{,}630{,}000 = m(300{,}000{,}000)^2$$
$$14{,}630{,}000 = m(90{,}000{,}000{,}000{,}000{,}000)$$
$$m = 0.000\ 000\ 000\ 163 \text{ kg}$$

I am not kidding; running 35 miles takes not even a couple thousandths of a millionth of a pound of body mass. 0.000 000 000 163 kg of body fat was converted into energy, which was literally converted to pure energy. What happened to the other 0.453 999 999 8 kg of body fat (the rest of the pound)? Don't worry; it's gone, too. It was converted to waste products (chemists like to call them combustion products) and eliminated from the body by one of two routes. And that is where this chapter ends – no pun intended.

APPENDIX A

Work Out / METs Tables

The best way to figure out how many Calories you are burning to do work is by using something called METs. MET stands for Metabolic EquivalenT. A MET is the number of Calories used to do work per minute of activity relative to the Basal Metabolic Rate (BMR). Most new exercise machines can display METs as well as Calories and are fairly accurate as long as you program in your correct weight.

A work out of 2-4 METs is considered light or mild exercise, 4-5 METs is considered moderate exercise, and more than 5 METs is considered vigorous exercise. Since METs are variable units depending on BMR you have to figure them out based on your body weight. Sound confusing? It's really not.

Take a look at the first page of the following table. The first activity is Aerobics - light. If you weigh 125 pounds, you will use or burn 3.0 Calories per minute. Exercise for 10 minutes and that's 30 (3.0 x 10) Calories. Exercise for 30 minutes and it's 90 (3.0 x 30) Calories.

Again, look at Aerobics - light. If you weigh 200 pounds, then each minute you're using 4.8 Calories. Ten minutes equal 48 Calories, and 30 minutes equal 144 Calories.

Try another one. You do 45 minutes of cycling at 10 mph and you weigh 175 pounds. What did you get? If you said 378 Calories (8.4 METs x 45 minutes), you're right!

One more? Okay, here's a tough one. You walk for 60 minutes and cover 3 miles, and you weigh 200 pounds. The answer ... 384 Calories. (3 miles in 60 minutes is 20 minutes per mile. In the table find 6.4 METs for a 200 pound person and then multiply by 60 minutes.)

If you fall in between weights, I recommend using the lower weight. You'll always be slightly underestimating the Calories used and therefore always slightly underestimating the weight you're losing. It's always better to step on the scale and be happily surprised to find that you actually lost more weight than you've figured you should have lost.

You can more precisely find the METs for any body weight, but it's more calculating. Do you see the third column that is just labeled METs? That's the column you need to look at. If you're up for it, here's the formula:

$$\text{METs} \times 3.5 \times \text{Body Weight in Pounds} \div 440$$

For example, if you weigh 160 pounds and run for 30 minutes at 12 minutes per mile pace, then you perform the following calculations:

$$8.7 \times 3.5 \times 160 \div 440 = 11.07 \text{ METs}$$

now multiply

$$11.07 \text{ METs} \times 30 \text{ minutes} = 332 \text{ Calories}$$

and you've done some serious calculating. Congratulations!

Activity	Intensity	METS	Cal per min at: 125 lb	150 lb	175 lb	200 lb	250 lb	300 lb
Aerobics	light	3.0	3.0	3.6	4.2	4.8	6.0	7.2
Aerobics	medium	6.0	6.0	7.2	8.4	9.5	11.9	14.3
Aerobics	hard	9.0	8.9	10.7	12.5	14.3	17.9	21.5
Archery	average	3.9	3.9	4.7	5.4	6.2	7.8	9.3
Backpacking	light	5.0	5.0	6.0	7.0	8.0	9.9	11.9
Backpacking	heavy	11.0	10.9	13.1	15.3	17.5	21.9	26.3
Badminton	low	4.0	4.0	4.8	5.6	6.4	8.0	9.5
Badminton	average	5.8	5.8	6.9	8.1	9.2	11.5	13.8
Badminton	high	9.0	8.9	10.7	12.5	14.3	17.9	21.5
Basketball	low	3.0	3.0	3.6	4.2	4.8	6.0	7.2
Basketball	non-game	4.0	4.0	4.8	5.6	6.4	8.0	9.5
Basketball	game	8.3	8.3	9.9	11.6	13.2	16.5	19.8
Basketball	high	12.0	11.9	14.3	16.7	19.1	23.9	28.6
Biking/ Bicycling	see Cycling							
Billiards		2.5	2.5	3.0	3.5	4.0	5.0	6.0
Bowling		3.5	3.5	4.2	4.9	5.6	7.0	8.4
Boxing	sparring	8.3	8.3	9.9	11.6	13.2	16.5	19.8
Boxing	kick boxing	9.0	8.9	10.7	12.5	14.3	17.9	21.5
Boxing	in-ring	13.3	13.2	15.9	18.5	21.2	26.2	31.7
Calisthenics	no weights	4.0	4.0	4.8	5.6	6.4	8.0	9.5
Canoeing	floating	3.0	3.0	3.6	4.2	4.8	6.0	7.2
Canoeing	leisure	4.0	4.0	4.8	5.6	6.4	8.0	9.5
Canoeing	medium	6.0	6.0	7.2	8.4	9.5	11.9	14.3
Canoeing	hard	8.0	8.0	9.5	11.1	12.7	15.9	19.1
Chopping Wood		5.0	5.0	6.0	7.0	8.0	9.9	11.9
Climbing Hills	low	5.0	5.0	6.0	7.0	8.0	9.9	11.9
Climbing Hills	average	7.2	7.2	8.6	10.0	11.5	14.3	17.2
Climbing Hills	high	10.0	9.9	11.9	13.9	15.9	19.9	23.9
Cricket	low	4.0	4.0	4.8	5.6	6.4	8.0	9.5
Cricket	average	5.2	5.2	6.2	7.2	8.3	10.3	12.4
Cricket	high	8.0	8.0	9.5	11.1	12.7	15.9	19.1
Croquet		3.5	3.5	4.2	4.9	5.6	7.0	8.4

Activity	Intensity	METS	Cal per min at: 125 lb	150 lb	175 lb	200 lb	250 lb	300 lb
Cutting Grass	self propelled	3.0	3.0	3.6	4.2	4.8	6.0	7.2
Cutting Grass	push mower	4.5	4.5	5.4	6.3	7.2	8.9	10.7
Cycling	6 mph	3.4	3.4	4.1	4.7	5.4	6.8	8.1
Cycling	7 mph	4.0	4.0	4.8	5.6	6.4	8.0	9.5
Cycling	10 mph	6.0	6.0	7.2	8.4	9.5	11.9	14.3
Cycling	12 mph	7.5	7.5	8.9	10.4	11.9	14.9	17.9
Cycling	15 mph	10.0	9.9	11.9	13.9	15.9	19.9	23.9
Cycling	20 mph	16.0	15.9	19.1	22.3	25.5	31.8	38.2
Dancing	social	4.0	4.0	4.8	5.6	6.4	8.0	9.5
Dancing	ballroom	4.5	4.5	5.4	6.3	7.2	8.9	10.7
Dancing	square	5.0	5.0	6.0	7.0	8.0	9.9	11.9
Dancing	ballet	6.0	6.0	7.2	8.4	9.5	11.9	14.3
Dancing	aerobic	7.0	7.0	8.4	9.7	11.1	13.9	16.7
Dancing	competitive	7.5	7.5	8.9	10.4	11.9	14.9	17.9
Driving	car	1.6	1.6	1.9	2.2	2.5	3.2	3.8
Fencing		8.0	8.0	9.5	11.1	12.7	15.9	19.1
Field Hockey		8.0	8.0	9.5	11.1	12.7	15.9	19.1
Fishing	sitting	2.0	2.0	2.4	2.8	3.2	4.0	4.8
Fishing	from bank	3.7	3.7	4.4	5.2	5.9	7.4	8.8
Fishing	wading	5.5	5.5	6.6	7.7	8.8	10.9	13.1
Football	touch	8.0	8.0	9.5	11.1	12.7	15.9	19.1
Gardening	no lifting	3.7	3.7	4.4	5.2	5.9	7.4	8.8
Golf	cart	2.3	2.3	2.7	3.2	3.7	4.6	5.5
Golf	walking	4.5	4.5	5.4	6.3	7.2	8.9	10.7
Handball		10.0	9.9	11.9	13.9	15.9	19.9	23.9
Horseback	walking	2.4	2.4	2.9	3.3	3.8	4.8	5.7
Horseback	trotting	6.6	6.6	7.9	9.2	10.5	13.1	15.8
Horseback	galloping	8.2	8.2	9.8	11.4	13.0	16.3	19.6
Horseshoes		2.5	2.5	3.0	3.5	4.0	5.0	6.0

Activity	Intensity	METS	Cal per min at: 125 lb	150 lb	175 lb	200 lb	250 lb	300 lb
Housework	light	2.5	2.5	3.0	3.5	4.0	5.0	6.0
Housework	watering	2.5	2.5	3.0	3.5	4.0	5.0	6.0
Housework	moderate	3.5	3.5	4.2	4.9	5.6	7.0	8.4
Housework	mopping	3.5	3.5	4.2	4.9	5.6	7.0	8.4
Housework	vacuuming	3.5	3.5	4.2	4.9	5.6	7.0	8.4
Housework	heavy	4.0	4.0	4.8	5.6	6.4	8.0	9.5
Hunting	walking - small game	5.0	5.0	6.0	7.0	8.0	9.9	11.9
Hunting	walking - big game	7.0	7.0	8.4	9.7	11.1	13.9	16.7
Jogging	see Running	about	100	Cal	per	mile		
Judo		13.5	13.5	16.1	18.8	21.5	26.8	32.2
Jumping Rope	60-80/min	9.0	8.9	10.7	12.5	14.3	17.9	21.5
Jumping Rope	80-120/min	10.5	10.4	12.5	14.6	16.7	20.9	25.1
Jumping Rope	120-140/min	11.0	10.9	13.1	15.3	17.5	21.9	26.3
Lawn Mower	power	3.0	3.0	3.6	4.2	4.8	6.0	7.2
Lawn Mower	push	4.5	4.5	5.4	6.3	7.2	8.9	10.7
Loading Car		3.0	3.0	3.6	4.2	4.8	6.0	7.2
Mountaineering	low	5.0	5.0	6.0	7.0	8.0	9.9	11.9
Mountaineering	high	10.0	9.9	11.9	13.9	15.9	19.9	23.9
Music	playing	2.5	2.5	3.0	3.5	4.0	5.0	6.0
Music	accordion	1.8	1.8	2.1	2.5	2.9	3.6	4.3
Music	cello	2.3	2.3	2.7	3.2	3.7	4.6	5.5
Music	flute	2.0	2.0	2.4	2.8	3.2	4.0	4.8
Music	piano	2.3	2.3	2.7	3.2	3.7	4.6	5.5
Music	violin	2.5	2.5	3.0	3.5	4.0	5.0	6.0
Ping Pong		4.0	4.0	4.8	5.6	6.4	8.0	9.5
Racquetball	low	8.0	8.0	9.5	11.1	12.7	15.9	19.1
Racquetball	average	9.0	8.9	10.7	12.5	14.3	17.9	21.5
Racquetball	high	12.0	11.9	14.3	16.7	19.1	23.9	28.9
Raking Lawn		4.0	4.0	4.8	5.6	6.4	8.0	9.5
Rock Climbing		10.0	9.9	11.9	13.9	15.9	19.9	23.9

Activity	Intensity	METS	Cal	per	min	at:		
			125 lb	150 lb	175 lb	200 lb	250 lb	300 lb
Rope Jumping	see Jumping	Rope						
Row Boat	slow-2.5 mph	3.0	3.0	3.6	4.2	4.8	6.0	7.2
Row Boat	medium	6.0	6.0	7.2	8.4	9.5	11.9	14.3
Row Boat	hard	8.0	8.0	9.5	11.1	12.7	15.9	19.1
Running	about	100	Cal	per	mile			
Running	12 min/mile	8.7	8.7	10.4	12.1	13.8	17.3	20.8
Running	11 min/mile	9.4	9.3	11.2	13.1	15.0	18.7	22.4
Running	10 min/mile	10.2	10.1	12.2	14.2	16.2	20.3	24.3
Running	9 min/mile	11.2	11.1	13.4	15.6	17.8	22.3	26.7
Running	8 min/mile	12.5	12.4	14.9	17.4	19.9	24.9	29.8
Running	7 min/mile	14.1	14.0	16.8	19.6	22.4	28.0	33.6
Running	6 min/mile	16.3	16.2	19.4	22.7	25.9	32.4	38.9
Sailing		3.5	3.5	4.2	4.9	5.6	7.0	8.4
Scuba Diving	low	5.0	5.0	6.0	7.0	8.0	9.9	11.9
Scuba Diving	average	7.5	7.5	8.9	10.4	11.9	14.9	17.9
Scuba Diving	high	10.0	9.9	11.9	13.9	15.9	19.9	23.9
Shopping		3.0	3.0	3.6	4.2	4.8	6.0	7.2
Shoveling		5.0	5.0	6.0	7.0	8.0	9.9	11.9
Shuffleboard		2.5	2.5	3.0	3.5	4.0	5.0	6.0
Sitting		1.4	1.4	1.7	1.9	2.2	2.8	3.3
Skating - ice/roller	low	5.0	5.0	6.0	7.0	8.0	9.9	11.9
Skating - ice/roller	10 mph	6.0	6.0	7.2	8.4	9.5	11.9	14.3
Skating - ice/roller	high	8.0	8.0	9.5	11.1	12.7	15.9	19.1
Skiing - downhill	low	5.0	5.0	6.0	7.0	8.0	9.9	11.9
Skiing - downhill	high	8.0	8.0	9.5	11.1	12.7	15.9	19.1

Activity	Intensity	METS	Cal per min at: 125 lb	150 lb	175 lb	200 lb	250 lb	300 lb
Skiing – water	low	5.0	5.0	6.0	7.0	8.0	9.9	11.9
Skiing – water	high	7.0	7.0	8.4	9.7	11.1	13.9	16.7
Skiing – xc	low	6.0	6.0	7.2	8.4	9.5	11.9	14.3
Skiing – xc	high	12.0	11.9	14.3	16.7	19.1	23.9	28.6
Sledding		6.0	6.0	7.2	8.4	9.5	11.9	14.3
Snowshoeing	easy	7.0	7.0	8.4	9.7	11.1	13.9	16.7
Snowshoeing	average	9.9	9.8	11.8	13.8	15.8	19.7	23.6
Snowshoeing	running	12.0	11.9	14.3	16.7	19.1	23.9	28.6
Soccer	non-game	5.0	5.0	6.0	7.0	8.0	9.9	11.9
Soccer	practice	8.0	8.0	9.5	11.1	12.7	15.9	19.1
Soccer	game	12.0	11.9	14.3	16.7	19.1	23.9	28.9
Squash	low	8.0	8.0	9.5	11.1	12.7	15.9	19.1
Squash	high	12.0	11.9	14.3	16.7	19.1	23.9	28.9
Surfing		6.0	6.0	7.2	8.4	9.5	11.9	14.3
Stairs	easy	4.0	4.0	4.8	5.6	6.4	8.0	9.5
Stairs	hard	8.0	8.0	9.5	11.1	12.7	15.9	19.1
Standing		2.0	2.0	2.4	2.8	3.2	4.0	4.8
Swimming	25 yds/min	3.8	3.8	4.5	5.3	6.0	7.6	9.1
Swimming	50 yds/min	7.0	7.0	8.4	9.7	11.1	13.9	16.7
Table Tennis		4.0	4.0	4.8	5.6	6.4	8.0	9.5
Taking out Trash		3.0	3.0	3.6	4.2	4.8	6.0	7.2
Tennis	doubles	5.5	5.5	6.6	7.7	8.8	10.9	13.1
Tennis	singles	6.5	6.5	7.8	9.0	10.3	12.9	15.5
Tennis	match play	9.0	8.9	10.7	12.5	14.3	17.9	21.5
Vacuuming		3.5	3.5	4.2	4.9	5.6	7.0	8.4
Volleyball	recrea-tional	3.0	3.0	3.6	4.2	4.8	6.0	7.2
Volleyball	competi-tive	6.0	6.0	7.2	8.4	9.5	11.9	14.3

Activity	Intensity	METS	Cal 125 lb	per 150 lb	min 175 lb	at: 200 lb	250 lb	300 lb
Walking	about	100	Cal	per	mile			
Walking	30 min/mile	3.0	3.0	3.6	4.2	4.8	6.0	7.2
Walking	20 min/mile	4.0	4.0	4.8	5.6	6.4	8.0	9.5
Walking	15 min/mile	5.2	5.2	6.2	7.2	8.3	10.3	12.4
Walking	12 min/mile	8.0	8.0	9.5	11.1	12.7	15.9	19.1
Walking	hills	7.5	7.5	8.9	10.4	11.9	14.9	17.9
Watering Plants		2.5	2.5	3.0	3.5	4.0	5.0	6.0
Water Skiing	low	5.0	5.0	6.0	7.0	8.0	9.9	11.9
Water Skiing	high	7.0	7.0	8.4	9.7	11.1	13.9	16.7
Work	desk	1.5	1.5	1.8	2.1	2.4	3.0	3.6
Yard Work	cut grass-power	3.0	3.0	3.6	4.2	4.8	6.0	7.2
Yard Work	gardening	3.7	3.7	4.4	5.2	5.9	7.4	8.8
Yard Work	raking	4.0	4.0	4.8	5.6	6.4	8.0	9.5
Yard Work	cut grass - push	4.5	4.5	5.4	6.3	7.2	8.9	10.7
Yard Work	shoveling	5.0	5.0	6.0	7.0	8.0	9.9	11.9

APPENDIX B

Calorie / kcal Tables

The following data table was provided by:
U.S. Department of Agriculture, Agricultural Research Service. 2002. USDA Nutrient Database for Standard Reference, Release 15. Nutrient Data Laboratory Home Page, http://www.nal.usda.gov/fnic/foodcomp.

The following pages may look hard to read, but there are only two columns you need to look at: "Measure of edible portion" and "Calories (kcal)." Measure of edible portion is just a fancy way of saying portion size (how much you ate) and Calories (kcal) is what I've been calling Energy In. Ignore all the other columns!

Take a look at the first item on the next page. Assuming you are 21 or older, if you drink a 12 oz. Regular beer you need to count 146 Calories. A 12 oz. Light beer only counts 99 Calories.

The table is divided into food groups. Be sure to highlight or mark the foods you usually eat.

You can also look at the food labels on the things you eat, but pay close attention to portion size. For example, no one I know only eats 1 oz. or 1 cup of breakfast cereal. A regular sized bowl can easily be 2-3 times that amount, which means you need to multiply the Calories by 2-3 as well. Many microwave popcorns list 3 servings per bag, but it seems about the right size just for me!

Table 9. Nutritive Value of the Edible Part of Food

Food No.	Food Description	Measure of edible portion	Weight (g)	Water (%)	Calories (kcal)	Protein (g)	Total fat (g)	Fatty acids		
								Saturated (g)	Monounsaturated (g)	Polyunsaturated (g)
	Beverages									
	Alcoholic									
	Beer									
1	Regular	12 fl oz	355	92	146	1	0	0.0	0.0	0.0
2	Light	12 fl oz	354	95	99	1	0	0.0	0.0	0.0
	Gin, rum, vodka, whiskey									
3	80 proof	1.5 fl oz	42	67	97	0	0	0.0	0.0	0.0
4	86 proof	1.5 fl oz	42	64	105	0	0	0.0	0.0	0.0
5	90 proof	1.5 fl oz	42	62	110	0	0	0.0	0.0	0.0
6	Liqueur, coffee, 53 proof	1.5 fl oz	52	31	175	Tr	Tr	0.1	Tr	0.1
	Mixed drinks, prepared from recipe									
7	Daiquiri	2 fl oz	60	70	112	Tr	Tr	Tr	Tr	Tr
8	Pina colada	4.5 fl oz	141	65	262	1	3	1.2	0.2	0.5
	Wine									
	Dessert									
9	Dry	3.5 fl oz	103	80	130	Tr	0	0.0	0.0	0.0
10	Sweet	3.5 fl oz	103	73	158	Tr	0	0.0	0.0	0.0
	Table									
11	Red	3.5 fl oz	103	89	74	Tr	0	0.0	0.0	0.0
12	White	3.5 fl oz	103	90	70	Tr	0	0.0	0.0	0.0
	Carbonated*									
13	Club soda	12 fl oz	355	100	0	0	0	0.0	0.0	0.0
14	Cola type	12 fl oz	370	89	152	0	0	0.0	0.0	0.0
	Diet, sweetened with aspartame									
15	Cola	12 fl oz	355	100	4	Tr	0	0.0	0.0	0.0
16	Other than cola or pepper type	12 fl oz	355	100	0	Tr	0	0.0	0.0	0.0
17	Ginger ale	12 fl oz	366	91	124	0	0	0.0	0.0	0.0
18	Grape	12 fl oz	372	89	160	0	0	0.0	0.0	0.0
19	Lemon lime	12 fl oz	368	90	147	0	0	0.0	0.0	0.0
20	Orange	12 fl oz	372	88	179	0	0	0.0	0.0	0.0
21	Pepper type	12 fl oz	368	89	151	0	Tr	0.3	0.0	0.0
22	Root beer	12 fl oz	370	89	152	0	0	0.0	0.0	0.0
	Chocolate flavored beverage mix									
23	Powder	2-3 heaping tsp	22	1	75	1	1	0.4	0.2	Tr
24	Prepared with milk	1 cup	266	81	226	9	9	5.5	2.6	0.3
	Cocoa									
	Powder containing nonfat dry milk									
25	Powder	3 heaping tsp	28	2	102	3	1	0.7	0.4	Tr
26	Prepared (6 oz water plus 1 oz powder)	1 serving	206	86	103	3	1	0.7	0.4	Tr
	Powder containing nonfat dry milk and aspartame									
27	Powder	½-oz envelope	15	3	48	4	Tr	0.3	0.1	Tr
28	Prepared (6 oz water plus 1 envelope mix)	1 serving	192	92	48	4	Tr	0.3	0.1	Tr
	Coffee									
29	Brewed	6 fl oz	178	99	4	Tr	0	Tr	0.0	Tr
30	Espresso	2 fl oz	60	98	5	Tr	Tr	0.1	0.0	0.1
31	Instant, prepared (1 rounded tsp powder plus 6 fl oz water)	6 fl oz	179	99	4	Tr	0	Tr	0.0	Tr

*Mineral content varies depending on water source.

Table 9. Nutritive Value of the Edible Part of Food

Food No.	Food Description	Measure of edible portion	Weight (g)	Water (%)	Calories (kcal)	Protein (g)	Total fat (g)	Fatty acids Saturated (g)	Fatty acids Monounsaturated (g)	Fatty acids Polyunsaturated (g)
	Beverages (continued)									
	Fruit drinks, noncarbonated, canned or bottled, with added ascorbic acid									
32	Cranberry juice cocktail	8 fl oz	253	86	144	0	Tr	Tr	Tr	0.1
33	Fruit punch drink	8 fl oz	248	88	117	0	0	Tr	Tr	Tr
34	Grape drink	8 fl oz	250	88	113	0	0	Tr	0.0	Tr
35	Pineapple grapefruit juice drink	8 fl oz	250	88	118	1	Tr	Tr	Tr	0.1
36	Pineapple orange juice drink	8 fl oz	250	87	125	3	0	0.0	0.0	0.0
	Lemonade									
37	Frozen concentrate, prepared	8 fl oz	248	89	99	Tr	0	Tr	Tr	Tr
	Powder, prepared with water									
38	Regular	8 fl oz	266	89	112	0	0	Tr	Tr	Tr
39	Low calorie, sweetened with aspartame	8 fl oz	237	99	5	0	0	0.0	0.0	0.0
	Malted milk, with added nutrients									
	Chocolate									
40	Powder	3 heaping tsp	21	3	75	1	1	0.4	0.2	0.1
41	Prepared	1 cup	265	81	225	9	9	5.5	2.6	0.4
	Natural									
42	Powder	4-5 heaping tsp	21	3	80	2	1	0.3	0.2	0.1
43	Prepared	1 cup	265	81	231	10	9	5.4	2.5	0.4
	Milk and milk beverages. See Dairy Products.									
44	Rice beverage, canned (RICE DREAM)	1 cup	245	89	120	Tr	2	0.2	1.3	0.3
	Soy milk. See Legumes, Nuts, and Seeds.									
	Tea									
	Brewed									
45	Black	6 fl oz	178	100	2	0	0	Tr	Tr	Tr
	Herb									
46	Chamomile	6 fl oz	178	100	2	0	0	Tr	Tr	Tr
47	Other than chamomile	6 fl oz	178	100	2	0	0	Tr	Tr	Tr
	Instant, powder, prepared									
48	Unsweetened	8 fl oz	237	100	2	0	0	0.0	0.0	0.0
49	Sweetened, lemon flavor	8 fl oz	259	91	88	Tr	0	Tr	Tr	Tr
50	Sweetened with saccharin, lemon flavor	8 fl oz	237	99	5	0	0	0.0	0.0	Tr
51	Water, tap	8 fl oz	237	100	0	0	0	0.0	0.0	0.0
	Dairy Products									
	Butter. See Fats and Oils.									
	Cheese									
	Natural									
52	Blue	1 oz	28	42	100	6	8	5.3	2.2	0.2
53	Camembert (3 wedges per 4-oz container)	1 wedge	38	52	114	8	9	5.8	2.7	0.3
	Cheddar									
54	Cut pieces	1 oz	28	37	114	7	9	6.0	2.7	0.3
55		1 cubic inch	17	37	68	4	6	3.6	1.6	0.2
56	Shredded	1 cup	113	37	455	28	37	23.8	10.6	1.1

Food No.	Food Description	Measure of edible portion	Weight (g)	Water (%)	Calories (kcal)	Protein (g)	Total fat (g)	Fatty acids: Saturated (g)	Fatty acids: Monounsaturated (g)	Fatty acids: Polyunsaturated (g)

Dairy Products (continued)

Food No.	Food Description	Measure of edible portion	Weight (g)	Water (%)	Calories (kcal)	Protein (g)	Total fat (g)	Saturated (g)	Monounsaturated (g)	Polyunsaturated (g)
	Cheese (continued)									
	Natural (continued)									
	Cottage									
	Creamed (4% fat)									
57	Large curd	1 cup	225	79	233	28	10	6.4	2.9	0.3
58	Small curd	1 cup	210	79	217	26	9	6.0	2.7	0.3
59	With fruit	1 cup	226	72	279	22	8	4.9	2.2	0.2
60	Low fat (2%)	1 cup	226	79	203	31	4	2.8	1.2	0.1
61	Low fat (1%)	1 cup	226	82	164	28	2	1.5	0.7	0.1
62	Uncreamed (dry curd, less than ½% fat)	1 cup	145	80	123	25	1	0.4	0.2	Tr
	Cream									
63	Regular	1 oz	28	54	99	2	10	6.2	2.8	0.4
64		1 tbsp	15	54	51	1	5	3.2	1.4	0.2
65	Low fat	1 tbsp	15	64	35	2	3	1.7	0.7	0.1
66	Fat free	1 tbsp	16	76	15	2	Tr	0.1	0.1	Tr
67	Feta	1 oz	28	55	75	4	6	4.2	1.3	0.2
68	Low fat, cheddar or colby	1 oz	28	63	49	7	2	1.2	0.6	0.1
	Mozzarella, made with									
69	Whole milk	1 oz	28	54	80	6	6	3.7	1.9	0.2
70	Part skim milk (low moisture)	1 oz	28	49	79	8	5	3.1	1.4	0.1
71	Muenster	1 oz	28	42	104	7	9	5.4	2.5	0.2
72	Neufchatel	1 oz	28	62	74	3	7	4.2	1.9	0.2
73	Parmesan, grated	1 cup	100	18	456	42	30	19.1	8.7	0.7
74		1 tbsp	5	18	23	2	2	1.0	0.4	Tr
75		1 oz	28	18	129	12	9	5.4	2.5	0.2
76	Provolone	1 oz	28	41	100	7	8	4.8	2.1	0.2
	Ricotta, made with									
77	Whole milk	1 cup	246	72	428	28	32	20.4	8.9	0.9
78	Part skim milk	1 cup	246	74	340	28	19	12.1	5.7	0.6
79	Swiss	1 oz	28	37	107	8	8	5.0	2.1	0.3
	Pasteurized process cheese									
	American									
80	Regular	1 oz	28	39	106	6	9	5.6	2.5	0.3
81	Fat free	1 slice	21	57	31	5	Tr	0.1	Tr	Tr
82	Swiss	1 oz	28	42	95	7	7	4.5	2.0	0.2
83	Pasteurized process cheese food, American	1 oz	28	43	93	6	7	4.4	2.0	0.2
84	Pasteurized process cheese spread, American	1 oz	28	48	82	5	6	3.8	1.8	0.2
	Cream, sweet									
85	Half and half (cream and milk)	1 cup	242	81	315	7	28	17.3	8.0	1.0
86		1 tbsp	15	81	20	Tr	2	1.1	0.5	0.1
87	Light, coffee, or table	1 cup	240	74	469	6	46	28.8	13.4	1.7
88		1 tbsp	15	74	29	Tr	3	1.8	0.8	0.1
	Whipping, unwhipped (volume about double when whipped)									
89	Light	1 cup	239	64	699	5	74	46.2	21.7	2.1
90		1 tbsp	15	64	44	Tr	5	2.9	1.4	0.1
91	Heavy	1 cup	238	58	821	5	88	54.8	25.4	3.3
92		1 tbsp	15	58	52	Tr	6	3.5	1.6	0.2
93	Whipped topping (pressurized)	1 cup	60	61	154	2	13	8.3	3.9	0.5
94		1 tbsp	3	61	8	Tr	1	0.4	0.2	Tr

Table 9. Nutritive Value of the Edible Part of Food

Food No.	Food Description	Measure of edible portion	Weight (g)	Water (%)	Calories (kcal)	Protein (g)	Total fat (g)	Fatty acids: Saturated (g)	Fatty acids: Monounsaturated (g)	Fatty acids: Polyunsaturated (g)
	Dairy Products (continued)									
	Cream, sour									
95	Regular	1 cup	230	71	493	7	48	30.0	13.9	1.8
96		1 tbsp	12	71	26	Tr	3	1.6	0.7	0.1
97	Reduced fat	1 tbsp	15	80	20	Tr	2	1.1	0.5	0.1
98	Fat free	1 tbsp	16	81	12	Tr	0	0.0	0.0	0.0
	Cream product, imitation (made with vegetable fat)									
	Sweet									
	Creamer									
99	Liquid (frozen)	1 tbsp	15	77	20	Tr	1	0.3	1.1	Tr
100	Powdered	1 tsp	2	2	11	Tr	1	0.7	Tr	Tr
	Whipped topping									
101	Frozen	1 cup	75	50	239	1	19	16.3	1.2	0.4
102		1 tbsp	4	50	13	Tr	1	0.9	0.1	Tr
103	Powdered, prepared with whole milk	1 cup	80	67	151	3	10	8.5	0.7	0.2
104		1 tbsp	4	67	8	Tr	Tr	0.4	Tr	Tr
105	Pressurized	1 cup	70	60	184	1	16	13.2	1.3	0.2
106		1 tbsp	4	60	11	Tr	1	0.8	0.1	Tr
107	Sour dressing (filled cream type, nonbutterfat)	1 cup	235	75	417	8	39	31.2	4.6	1.1
108		1 tbsp	12	75	21	Tr	2	1.6	0.2	0.1
	Frozen dessert									
	Frozen yogurt, soft serve									
109	Chocolate	½ cup	72	64	115	3	4	2.6	1.3	0.2
110	Vanilla	½ cup	72	65	114	3	4	2.5	1.1	0.2
	Ice cream									
	Regular									
111	Chocolate	½ cup	66	56	143	3	7	4.5	2.1	0.3
112	Vanilla	½ cup	66	61	133	2	7	4.5	2.1	0.3
113	Light (50% reduced fat), vanilla	½ cup	66	68	92	3	3	1.7	0.8	0.1
114	Premium low fat, chocolate	½ cup	72	61	113	3	2	1.0	0.6	0.1
115	Rich, vanilla	½ cup	74	57	178	3	12	7.4	3.4	0.4
116	Soft serve, french vanilla	½ cup	86	60	185	4	11	6.4	3.0	0.4
117	Sherbet, orange	½ cup	74	66	102	1	1	0.9	0.4	0.1
	Milk									
	Fluid, no milk solids added									
118	Whole (3.3% fat)	1 cup	244	88	150	8	8	5.1	2.4	0.3
119	Reduced fat (2%)	1 cup	244	89	121	8	5	2.9	1.4	0.2
120	Lowfat (1%)	1 cup	244	90	102	8	3	1.6	0.7	0.1
121	Nonfat (skim)	1 cup	245	91	86	8	Tr	0.3	0.1	Tr
122	Buttermilk	1 cup	245	90	99	8	2	1.3	0.6	0.1
	Canned									
123	Condensed, sweetened	1 cup	306	27	982	24	27	16.8	7.4	1.0
	Evaporated									
124	Whole milk	1 cup	252	74	339	17	19	11.6	5.9	0.6
125	Skim milk	1 cup	256	79	199	19	1	0.3	0.2	Tr
	Dried									
126	Buttermilk	1 cup	120	3	464	41	7	4.3	2.0	0.3
127	Nonfat, instant, with added vitamin A	1 cup	68	4	244	24	Tr	0.3	0.1	Tr
	Milk beverage									
	Chocolate milk (commercial)									
128	Whole	1 cup	250	82	208	8	8	5.3	2.5	0.3
129	Reduced fat (2%)	1 cup	250	84	179	8	5	3.1	1.5	0.2
130	Lowfat (1%)	1 cup	250	85	158	8	3	1.5	0.8	0.1

*The vitamin A values listed for imitation sweet cream products are mostly from beta-carotene added for coloring.

Table 9. Nutritive Value of the Edible Part of Food

Food No.	Food Description	Measure of edible portion	Weight (g)	Water (%)	Calories (kcal)	Protein (g)	Total fat (g)	Fatty acids Saturated (g)	Fatty acids Monounsaturated (g)	Fatty acids Polyunsaturated (g)

Dairy Products (continued)

Food No.	Food Description	Measure of edible portion	Weight (g)	Water (%)	Calories (kcal)	Protein (g)	Total fat (g)	Saturated (g)	Monounsaturated (g)	Polyunsaturated (g)
	Milk beverage (continued)									
131	Eggnog (commercial)	1 cup	254	74	342	10	19	11.3	5.7	0.9
	Milk shake, thick									
132	Chocolate	10.6 fl oz	300	72	356	9	8	5.0	2.3	0.3
133	Vanilla	11 fl oz	313	74	350	12	9	5.9	2.7	0.4
	Sherbet. See Dairy Products, frozen dessert.									
	Yogurt									
	With added milk solids									
	Made with lowfat milk									
134	Fruit flavored	8-oz container	227	74	231	10	2	1.6	0.7	0.1
135	Plain	8-oz container	227	85	144	12	4	2.3	1.0	0.1
	Made with nonfat milk									
136	Fruit flavored	8-oz container	227	75	213	10	Tr	0.3	0.1	Tr
137	Plain	8-oz container	227	85	127	13	Tr	0.3	0.1	Tr
	Without added milk solids									
138	Made with whole milk, plain	8-oz container	227	88	139	8	7	4.8	2.0	0.2
139	Made with nonfat milk, low calorie sweetener, vanilla or lemon flavor	8-oz container	227	87	98	9	Tr	0.3	0.1	Tr

Eggs

Food No.	Food Description	Measure of edible portion	Weight (g)	Water (%)	Calories (kcal)	Protein (g)	Total fat (g)	Saturated (g)	Monounsaturated (g)	Polyunsaturated (g)
	Egg									
	Raw									
140	Whole	1 medium	44	75	66	5	4	1.4	1.7	0.6
141		1 large	50	75	75	6	5	1.6	1.9	0.7
142		1 extra large	58	75	86	7	6	1.8	2.2	0.8
143	White	1 large	33	88	17	4	0	0.0	0.0	0.0
144	Yolk	1 large	17	49	59	3	5	1.6	1.9	0.7
	Cooked, whole									
145	Fried, in margarine, with salt	1 large	46	69	92	6	7	1.9	2.7	1.3
146	Hard cooked, shell removed	1 large	50	75	78	6	5	1.6	2.0	0.7
147		1 cup, chopped	136	75	211	17	14	4.4	5.5	1.9
148	Poached, with salt	1 large	50	75	75	6	5	1.5	1.9	0.7
149	Scrambled, in margarine, with whole milk, salt	1 large	61	73	101	7	7	2.2	2.9	1.3
150	Egg substitute, liquid	¼ cup	63	83	53	8	2	0.4	0.6	1.0

Fats and Oils

Food No.	Food Description	Measure of edible portion	Weight (g)	Water (%)	Calories (kcal)	Protein (g)	Total fat (g)	Saturated (g)	Monounsaturated (g)	Polyunsaturated (g)
	Butter (4 sticks per lb)									
151	Salted	1 stick	113	16	813	1	92	57.3	26.6	3.4
152		1 tbsp	14	16	102	Tr	12	7.2	3.3	0.4
153		1 tsp	5	16	36	Tr	4	2.5	1.2	0.2
154	Unsalted	1 stick	113	18	813	1	92	57.3	26.6	3.4
155	Lard	1 cup	205	0	1,849	0	205	80.4	92.5	23.0
156		1 tbsp	13	0	115	0	13	5.0	5.8	1.4
	Margarine, vitamin A-fortified, salt added									
	Regular (about 80% fat)									
157	Hard (4 sticks per lb)	1 stick	113	16	815	1	91	17.9	40.6	28.8
158		1 tbsp	14	16	101	Tr	11	2.2	5.0	3.6
159		1 tsp	5	16	34	Tr	4	0.7	1.7	1.2
160	Soft	1 cup	227	16	1,626	2	183	31.3	64.7	78.5
161		1 tsp	5	16	34	Tr	4	0.6	1.3	1.6

Fats and Oils (continued)

Food No.	Food Description	Measure of edible portion	Weight (g)	Water (%)	Calories (kcal)	Protein (g)	Total fat (g)	Fatty acids: Saturated (g)	Fatty acids: Monounsaturated (g)	Fatty acids: Polyunsaturated (g)
	Margarine, vitamin A-fortified, salt added (continued)									
	Spread (about 60% fat)									
162	Hard (4 sticks per lb)	1 stick	115	37	621	1	70	16.2	29.9	20.8
163		1 tbsp	14	37	76	Tr	9	2.0	3.6	2.5
164		1 tsp	5	37	26	Tr	3	0.7	1.2	0.9
165	Soft	1 cup	229	37	1,236	1	139	29.3	72.1	31.6
166		1 tsp	5	37	26	Tr	3	0.6	1.5	0.7
167	Spread (about 40% fat)	1 cup	232	58	801	1	90	17.9	36.4	32.0
168		1 tsp	5	58	17	Tr	2	0.4	0.8	0.7
169	Margarine butter blend	1 stick	113	16	811	1	91	32.1	37.0	18.0
170		1 tbsp	14	16	102	Tr	11	4.0	4.7	2.3
	Oils, salad or cooking									
171	Canola	1 cup	218	0	1,927	0	218	15.5	128.4	64.5
172		1 tbsp	14	0	124	0	14	1.0	8.2	4.1
173	Corn	1 cup	218	0	1,927	0	218	27.7	52.8	128.0
174		1 tbsp	14	0	120	0	14	1.7	3.3	8.0
175	Olive	1 cup	216	0	1,909	0	216	29.2	159.2	18.1
176		1 tbsp	14	0	119	0	14	1.8	9.9	1.1
177	Peanut	1 cup	216	0	1,909	0	216	36.5	99.8	69.1
178		1 tbsp	14	0	119	0	14	2.3	6.2	4.3
179	Safflower, high oleic	1 cup	218	0	1,927	0	218	13.5	162.7	31.3
180		1 tbsp	14	0	120	0	14	0.8	10.2	2.0
181	Sesame	1 cup	218	0	1,927	0	218	31.0	86.5	90.9
182		1 tbsp	14	0	120	0	14	1.9	5.4	5.7
183	Soybean, hydrogenated	1 cup	218	0	1,927	0	218	32.5	93.7	82.0
184		1 tbsp	14	0	120	0	14	2.0	5.8	5.1
185	Soybean, hydrogenated and cottonseed oil blend	1 cup	218	0	1,927	0	218	39.2	64.3	104.9
186		1 tbsp	14	0	120	0	14	2.4	4.0	6.5
187	Sunflower	1 cup	218	0	1,927	0	218	22.5	42.5	143.2
188		1 tbsp	14	0	120	0	14	1.4	2.7	8.9
	Salad dressings									
	Commercial									
	Blue cheese									
189	Regular	1 tbsp	15	32	77	1	8	1.5	1.9	4.3
190	Low calorie	1 tbsp	15	80	15	1	1	0.4	0.3	0.4
	Caesar									
191	Regular	1 tbsp	15	34	78	Tr	8	1.3	2.0	4.8
192	Low calorie	1 tbsp	15	73	17	Tr	1	0.1	0.2	0.4
	French									
193	Regular	1 tbsp	16	38	67	Tr	6	1.5	1.2	3.4
194	Low calorie	1 tbsp	16	69	22	Tr	1	0.1	0.2	0.6
	Italian									
195	Regular	1 tbsp	15	38	69	Tr	7	1.0	1.6	4.1
196	Low calorie	1 tbsp	15	82	16	Tr	1	0.2	0.3	0.9
	Mayonnaise									
197	Regular	1 tbsp	14	15	99	Tr	11	1.6	3.1	5.7
198	Light, cholesterol free	1 tbsp	15	56	49	Tr	5	0.7	1.1	2.8
199	Fat free	1 tbsp	16	84	12	0	Tr	0.1	0.1	0.2
	Russian									
200	Regular	1 tbsp	15	35	76	Tr	8	1.1	1.8	4.5
201	Low calorie	1 tbsp	16	65	23	Tr	1	0.1	0.1	0.4
	Thousand island									
202	Regular	1 tbsp	16	46	59	Tr	6	0.9	1.3	3.1
203	Low calorie	1 tbsp	15	69	24	Tr	2	0.2	0.4	0.9

Table 9. Nutritive Value of the Edible Part of Food

Fats and Oils (continued)

Food No.	Food Description	Measure of edible portion	Weight (g)	Water (%)	Calories (kcal)	Protein (g)	Total fat (g)	Fatty acids: Saturated (g)	Fatty acids: Monounsaturated (g)	Fatty acids: Polyunsaturated (g)
	Salad dressings (continued)									
	Prepared from home recipe									
204	Cooked, made with margarine	1 tbsp	16	69	25	1	2	0.5	0.6	0.3
205	French	1 tbsp	14	24	88	Tr	10	1.8	2.9	4.7
206	Vinegar and oil	1 tbsp	16	47	70	0	8	1.4	2.3	3.8
207	Shortening (hydrogenated soybean and cottonseed oils)	1 cup	205	0	1,812	0	205	51.3	91.2	53.5
208		1 tbsp	13	0	113	0	13	3.2	5.7	3.3

Fish and Shellfish

Food No.	Food Description	Measure of edible portion	Weight (g)	Water (%)	Calories (kcal)	Protein (g)	Total fat (g)	Fatty acids: Saturated (g)	Fatty acids: Monounsaturated (g)	Fatty acids: Polyunsaturated (g)
209	Catfish, breaded, fried	3 oz	85	59	195	15	11	2.8	4.8	2.8
	Clam									
210	Raw, meat only	3 oz	85	82	63	11	1	0.1	0.1	0.2
211		1 medium	15	82	11	2	Tr	Tr	Tr	Tr
212	Breaded, fried	¾ cup	115	29	451	13	26	6.6	11.4	6.8
213	Canned, drained solids	3 oz	85	64	126	22	2	0.2	0.1	0.5
214		1 cup	160	64	237	41	3	0.3	0.3	0.9
	Cod									
215	Baked or broiled	3 oz	85	76	89	20	1	0.1	0.1	0.3
216		1 fillet	90	76	95	21	1	0.1	0.1	0.3
217	Canned, solids and liquid	3 oz	85	76	89	19	1	0.1	0.1	0.2
	Crab									
	Alaska king									
218	Steamed	1 leg	134	78	130	26	2	0.2	0.2	0.7
219		3 oz	85	78	82	16	1	0.1	0.2	0.5
220	Imitation, from surimi	3 oz	85	74	87	10	1	0.2	0.2	0.6
	Blue									
221	Steamed	3 oz	85	77	87	17	2	0.2	0.2	0.6
222	Canned crabmeat	1 cup	135	76	134	28	2	0.3	0.3	0.6
223	Crab cake, with egg, onion, fried in margarine	1 cake	60	71	93	12	5	0.9	1.7	1.4
224	Fish fillet, battered or breaded, fried	1 fillet	91	54	211	13	11	2.6	2.3	5.7
225	Fish stick and portion, breaded, frozen, reheated	1 stick (4" x 1" x ½")	28	46	76	4	3	0.9	1.4	0.9
226		1 portion (4" x 2" x ½")	57	46	155	9	7	1.8	2.9	1.8
227	Flounder or sole, baked or broiled	3 oz	85	73	99	21	1	0.3	0.2	0.5
228		1 fillet	127	73	149	31	2	0.5	0.3	0.8
229	Haddock, baked or broiled	3 oz	85	74	95	21	1	0.1	0.1	0.3
230		1 fillet	150	74	168	36	1	0.3	0.2	0.5
231	Halibut, baked or broiled	3 oz	85	72	119	23	2	0.4	0.8	0.8
232		½ fillet	159	72	223	42	5	0.7	1.5	1.5
233	Herring, pickled	3 oz	85	55	223	12	15	2.0	10.2	1.4
234	Lobster, steamed	3 oz	85	76	83	17	1	0.1	0.1	0.1
235	Ocean perch, baked or broiled	3 oz	85	73	103	20	2	0.3	0.7	0.5
236		1 fillet	50	73	61	12	1	0.2	0.4	0.3
	Oyster									
237	Raw, meat only	1 cup	248	85	169	17	6	1.9	0.8	2.4
238		6 medium	84	85	57	6	2	0.6	0.3	0.8
239	Breaded, fried	3 oz	85	65	167	7	11	2.7	4.0	2.8
240	Pollock, baked or broiled	3 oz	85	74	96	20	1	0.2	0.1	0.4
241		1 fillet	60	74	68	14	1	0.1	0.1	0.3
242	Rockfish, baked or broiled	3 oz	85	73	103	20	2	0.4	0.4	0.5
243		1 fillet	149	73	180	36	3	0.7	0.7	0.9

Food No.	Food Description	Measure of edible portion	Weight (g)	Water (%)	Calories (kcal)	Protein (g)	Total fat (g)	Fatty acids: Saturated (g)	Fatty acids: Monounsaturated (g)	Fatty acids: Polyunsaturated (g)

Fish and Shellfish (continued)

Food No.	Food Description	Measure of edible portion	Weight (g)	Water (%)	Calories (kcal)	Protein (g)	Total fat (g)	Saturated (g)	Monounsaturated (g)	Polyunsaturated (g)
244	Roughy, orange, baked or broiled	3 oz	85	69	76	16	1	Tr	0.5	Tr
	Salmon									
245	Baked or broiled (red)	3 oz	85	62	184	23	9	1.6	4.5	2.0
246		½ fillet	155	62	335	42	17	3.0	8.2	3.7
247	Canned (pink), solids and liquid (includes bones)	3 oz	85	69	118	17	5	1.3	1.5	1.7
248	Smoked (chinook)	3 oz	85	72	99	16	4	0.8	1.7	0.8
249	Sardine, Atlantic, canned in oil, drained solids (includes bones)	3 oz	85	60	177	21	10	1.3	3.3	4.4
	Scallop, cooked									
250	Breaded, fried	6 large	93	58	200	17	10	2.5	4.2	2.7
251	Steamed	3 oz	85	73	95	20	1	0.1	0.1	0.4
	Shrimp									
252	Breaded, fried	3 oz	85	53	206	18	10	1.8	3.2	4.3
253		6 large	45	53	109	10	6	0.9	1.7	2.3
254	Canned, drained solids	3 oz	85	73	102	20	2	0.3	0.2	0.6
255	Swordfish, baked or broiled	3 oz	85	69	132	22	4	1.2	1.7	1.0
256		1 piece	106	69	164	27	5	1.5	2.1	1.3
257	Trout, baked or broiled	3 oz	85	68	144	21	6	1.8	1.8	2.0
258		1 fillet	71	68	120	17	5	1.5	1.5	1.7
	Tuna									
259	Baked or broiled	3 oz	85	63	118	25	1	0.3	0.2	0.3
	Canned, drained solids									
260	Oil pack, chunk light	3 oz	85	60	168	25	7	1.3	2.5	2.5
261	Water pack, chunk light	3 oz	85	75	99	22	1	0.2	0.1	0.3
262	Water pack, solid white	3 oz	85	73	109	20	3	0.7	0.7	0.9
263	Tuna salad: light tuna in oil, pickle relish, mayo type salad dressing	1 cup	205	63	383	33	19	3.2	5.9	8.5

Fruits and Fruit Juices

Food No.	Food Description	Measure of edible portion	Weight (g)	Water (%)	Calories (kcal)	Protein (g)	Total fat (g)	Saturated (g)	Monounsaturated (g)	Polyunsaturated (g)
	Apples									
	Raw									
264	Unpeeled, 2¾" dia (about 3 per lb)	1 apple	138	84	81	Tr	Tr	0.1	Tr	0.1
265	Peeled, sliced	1 cup	110	84	63	Tr	Tr	0.1	Tr	0.1
266	Dried (sodium bisulfite used to preserve color)	5 rings	32	32	78	Tr	Tr	Tr	Tr	Tr
267	Apple juice, bottled or canned	1 cup	248	88	117	Tr	Tr	Tr	Tr	0.1
268	Apple pie filling, canned	⅛ of 21-oz can	74	73	75	Tr	Tr	Tr	0.0	Tr
	Applesauce, canned									
269	Sweetened	1 cup	255	80	194	Tr	Tr	0.1	Tr	0.1
270	Unsweetened	1 cup	244	88	105	Tr	Tr	Tr	Tr	Tr
	Apricots									
271	Raw, without pits (about 12 per lb with pits)	1 apricot	35	86	17	Tr	Tr	Tr	0.1	Tr
	Canned, halves, fruit and liquid									
272	Heavy syrup pack	1 cup	258	78	214	1	Tr	Tr	0.1	Tr
273	Juice pack	1 cup	244	87	117	2	Tr	Tr	Tr	Tr
274	Dried, sulfured	10 halves	35	31	83	1	Tr	Tr	0.1	Tr
275	Apricot nectar, canned, with added ascorbic acid	1 cup	251	85	141	1	Tr	Tr	0.1	Tr
	Asian pear, raw									
276	2¼" high x 2½" dia	1 pear	122	88	51	1	Tr	Tr	0.1	0.1
277	3⅜" high x 3" dia	1 pear	275	88	116	1	1	Tr	0.1	0.2

Table 9. Nutritive Value of the Edible Part of Food

Food No.	Food Description	Measure of edible portion	Weight (g)	Water (%)	Calories (kcal)	Protein (g)	Total fat (g)	Fatty acids Saturated (g)	Fatty acids Monounsaturated (g)	Fatty acids Polyunsaturated (g)

Fruits and Fruit Juices (continued)

Food No.	Food Description	Measure of edible portion	Weight (g)	Water (%)	Calories (kcal)	Protein (g)	Total fat (g)	Saturated (g)	Monounsaturated (g)	Polyunsaturated (g)
	Avocados, raw, without skin and seed									
278	California (about ⅕ whole)	1 oz	28	73	50	1	5	0.7	3.2	0.6
279	Florida (about 1/10 whole)	1 oz	28	80	32	Tr	3	0.5	1.4	0.4
	Bananas, raw									
280	Whole, medium (7" to 7⅞" long)	1 banana	118	74	109	1	1	0.2	Tr	0.1
281	Sliced	1 cup	150	74	138	2	1	0.3	0.1	0.1
282	Blackberries, raw	1 cup	144	86	75	1	1	Tr	0.1	0.3
	Blueberries									
283	Raw	1 cup	145	85	81	1	1	Tr	0.1	0.2
284	Frozen, sweetened, thawed	1 cup	230	77	186	1	Tr	Tr	Tr	0.1
	Cantaloupe. See Melons.									
	Carambola (starfruit), raw									
285	Whole (3⅝" long)	1 fruit	91	91	30	Tr	Tr	Tr	Tr	0.2
286	Sliced	1 cup	108	91	36	1	Tr	Tr	Tr	0.2
	Cherries									
287	Sour, red, pitted, canned, water pack	1 cup	244	90	88	2	Tr	0.1	0.1	0.1
288	Sweet, raw, without pits and stems	10 cherries	68	81	49	1	1	0.1	0.2	0.2
289	Cherry pie filling, canned	⅕ of 21-oz can	74	71	85	Tr	Tr	Tr	Tr	Tr
290	Cranberries, dried, sweetened	¼ cup	28	12	92	Tr	Tr	Tr	Tr	0.1
291	Cranberry sauce, sweetened, canned (about 8 slices per can)	1 slice	57	61	86	Tr	Tr	Tr	Tr	Tr
	Dates, without pits									
292	Whole	5 dates	42	23	116	1	Tr	0.1	0.1	Tr
293	Chopped	1 cup	178	23	490	4	1	0.3	0.3	0.1
294	Figs, dried	2 figs	38	28	97	1	Tr	0.1	0.1	0.2
	Fruit cocktail, canned, fruit and liquid									
295	Heavy syrup pack	1 cup	248	80	181	1	Tr	Tr	Tr	0.1
296	Juice pack	1 cup	237	87	109	1	Tr	Tr	Tr	Tr
	Grapefruit									
	Raw, without peel, membrane and seeds (3¾" dia)									
297	Pink or red	½ grapefruit	123	91	37	1	Tr	Tr	Tr	Tr
298	White	½ grapefruit	118	90	39	1	Tr	Tr	Tr	Tr
299	Canned, sections with light syrup	1 cup	254	84	152	1	Tr	Tr	Tr	0.1
	Grapefruit juice									
	Raw									
300	Pink	1 cup	247	90	96	1	Tr	Tr	Tr	0.1
301	White	1 cup	247	90	96	1	Tr	Tr	Tr	0.1
	Canned									
302	Unsweetened	1 cup	247	90	94	1	Tr	Tr	Tr	0.1
303	Sweetened	1 cup	250	87	115	1	Tr	Tr	Tr	0.1
	Frozen concentrate, unsweetened									
304	Undiluted	6-fl-oz can	207	62	302	4	1	0.1	0.1	0.2
305	Diluted with 3 parts water by volume	1 cup	247	89	101	1	Tr	Tr	Tr	0.1
306	Grapes, seedless, raw	10 grapes	50	81	36	Tr	Tr	0.1	Tr	0.1
307		1 cup	160	81	114	1	1	0.3	Tr	0.3

Fruits and Fruit Juices (continued)

Food No.	Food Description	Measure of edible portion	Weight (g)	Water (%)	Calories (kcal)	Protein (g)	Total fat (g)	Fatty acids: Saturated (g)	Fatty acids: Monounsaturated (g)	Fatty acids: Polyunsaturated (g)
	Grape juice									
308	Canned or bottled	1 cup	253	84	154	1	Tr	0.1	Tr	0.1
	Frozen concentrate, sweetened, with added vitamin C									
309	Undiluted	6-fl-oz can	216	54	387	1	1	0.2	Tr	0.2
310	Diluted with 3 parts water by volume	1 cup	250	87	128	Tr	Tr	0.1	Tr	0.1
311	Kiwi fruit, raw, without skin (about 5 per lb with skin)	1 medium	76	83	46	1	Tr	Tr	Tr	0.2
312	Lemons, raw, without peel (2⅛" dia with peel)	1 lemon	58	89	17	1	Tr	Tr	Tr	0.1
	Lemon juice									
313	Raw (from 2⅛"-dia lemon)	juice of 1 lemon	47	91	12	Tr	0	0.0	0.0	0.0
314	Canned or bottled, unsweetened	1 cup	244	92	51	1	1	0.1	Tr	0.2
315		1 tbsp	15	92	3	Tr	Tr	Tr	Tr	Tr
	Lime juice									
316	Raw (from 2"-dia lime)	juice of 1 lime	38	90	10	Tr	Tr	Tr	Tr	Tr
317	Canned, unsweetened	1 cup	246	93	52	1	1	0.1	0.1	0.2
318		1 tbsp	15	93	3	Tr	Tr	Tr	Tr	Tr
	Mangos, raw, without skin and seed (about 1½ per lb with skin and seed)									
319	Whole	1 mango	207	82	135	1	1	0.1	0.2	0.1
320	Sliced	1 cup	165	82	107	1	Tr	0.1	0.2	0.1
	Melons, raw, without rind and cavity contents									
	Cantaloupe (5" dia)									
321	Wedge	⅛ melon	69	90	24	1	Tr	Tr	Tr	0.1
322	Cubes	1 cup	160	90	56	1	Tr	0.1	Tr	0.2
	Honeydew (6"-7" dia)									
323	Wedge	⅛ melon	160	90	56	1	Tr	Tr	Tr	0.1
324	Diced (about 20 pieces per cup)	1 cup	170	90	60	1	Tr	Tr	Tr	0.1
325	Mixed fruit, frozen, sweetened, thawed (peach, cherry, raspberry, grape and boysenberry)	1 cup	250	74	245	4	Tr	0.1	0.1	0.2
326	Nectarines, raw (2½" dia)	1 nectarine	136	86	67	1	1	0.1	0.2	0.3
	Oranges, raw									
327	Whole, without peel and seeds (2⅝" dia)	1 orange	131	87	62	1	Tr	Tr	Tr	Tr
328	Sections without membranes	1 cup	180	87	85	2	Tr	Tr	Tr	Tr
	Orange juice									
329	Raw, all varieties	1 cup	248	88	112	2	Tr	0.1	0.1	0.1
330		juice from 1 orange	86	88	39	1	Tr	Tr	Tr	Tr
331	Canned, unsweetened	1 cup	249	89	105	1	Tr	Tr	0.1	0.1
332	Chilled (refrigerator case)	1 cup	249	88	110	2	1	0.1	0.1	0.2
	Frozen concentrate									
333	Undiluted	6-fl-oz can	213	58	339	5	Tr	0.1	0.1	0.1
334	Diluted with 3 parts water by volume	1 cup	249	88	112	2	Tr	Tr	Tr	Tr
	Papayas, raw									
335	½" cubes	1 cup	140	89	55	1	Tr	0.1	0.1	Tr
336	Whole (5⅛" long x 3" dia)	1 papaya	304	89	119	2	Tr	0.1	0.1	0.1

*Sodium benzoate and sodium bisulfite added as preservatives.

Food No.	Food Description	Measure of edible portion	Weight (g)	Water (%)	Calories (kcal)	Protein (g)	Total fat (g)	Fatty acids: Saturated (g)	Fatty acids: Monounsaturated (g)	Fatty acids: Polyunsaturated (g)

Fruits and Fruit Juices (continued)

Food No.	Food Description	Measure of edible portion	Weight (g)	Water (%)	Calories (kcal)	Protein (g)	Total fat (g)	Saturated (g)	Monounsaturated (g)	Polyunsaturated (g)
	Peaches									
	Raw									
337	Whole, 2½" dia, pitted (about 4 per lb)	1 peach	98	88	42	1	Tr	Tr	Tr	Tr
338	Sliced	1 cup	170	88	73	1	Tr	Tr	0.1	0.1
	Canned, fruit and liquid									
339	Heavy syrup pack	1 cup	262	79	194	1	Tr	Tr	0.1	0.1
340		1 half	98	79	73	Tr	Tr	Tr	Tr	Tr
341	Juice pack	1 cup	248	87	109	2	Tr	Tr	Tr	Tr
342		1 half	98	87	43	1	Tr	Tr	Tr	Tr
343	Dried, sulfured	3 halves	39	32	93	1	Tr	Tr	0.1	0.1
344	Frozen, sliced, sweetened, with added ascorbic acid, thawed	1 cup	250	75	235	2	Tr	Tr	0.1	0.2
	Pears									
345	Raw, with skin, cored, 2½" dia	1 pear	166	84	98	1	1	Tr	0.1	0.2
	Canned, fruit and liquid									
346	Heavy syrup pack	1 cup	266	80	197	1	Tr	Tr	0.1	0.1
347		1 half	76	80	56	Tr	Tr	Tr	Tr	Tr
348	Juice pack	1 cup	248	86	124	1	Tr	Tr	Tr	Tr
349		1 half	76	86	38	Tr	Tr	Tr	Tr	Tr
	Pineapple									
350	Raw, diced	1 cup	155	87	76	1	1	Tr	0.1	0.2
	Canned, fruit and liquid									
	Heavy syrup pack									
351	Crushed, sliced, or chunks	1 cup	254	79	198	1	Tr	Tr	Tr	0.1
352	Slices (3" dia)	1 slice	49	79	38	Tr	Tr	Tr	Tr	Tr
	Juice pack									
353	Crushed, sliced, or chunks	1 cup	249	84	149	1	Tr	Tr	Tr	0.1
354	Slice (3" dia)	1 slice	47	84	28	Tr	Tr	Tr	Tr	Tr
355	Pineapple juice, unsweetened, canned	1 cup	250	86	140	1	Tr	Tr	Tr	0.1
	Plantain, without peel									
356	Raw	1 medium	179	65	218	2	1	0.3	0.1	0.1
357	Cooked, slices	1 cup	154	67	179	1	Tr	0.1	Tr	0.1
	Plums									
358	Raw (2⅛" dia)	1 plum	66	85	36	1	Tr	Tr	0.3	0.1
	Canned, purple, fruit and liquid									
359	Heavy syrup pack	1 cup	258	76	230	1	Tr	Tr	0.2	0.1
360		1 plum	46	76	41	Tr	Tr	Tr	Tr	Tr
361	Juice pack	1 cup	252	84	146	1	Tr	Tr	Tr	Tr
362		1 plum	46	84	27	Tr	Tr	Tr	Tr	Tr
	Prunes, dried, pitted									
363	Uncooked	5 prunes	42	32	100	1	Tr	Tr	0.1	Tr
364	Stewed, unsweetened, fruit and liquid	1 cup	248	70	265	3	1	Tr	0.4	0.1
365	Prune juice, canned or bottled	1 cup	256	81	182	2	Tr	Tr	0.1	Tr
	Raisins, seedless									
366	Cup, not packed	1 cup	145	15	435	5	1	0.2	Tr	0.2
367	Packet, ½ oz (1½ tbsp)	1 packet	14	15	42	Tr	Tr	Tr	Tr	Tr
	Raspberries									
368	Raw	1 cup	123	87	60	1	1	Tr	0.1	0.4
369	Frozen, sweetened, thawed	1 cup	250	73	258	2	Tr	Tr	Tr	0.2
370	Rhubarb, frozen, cooked, with sugar	1 cup	240	68	278	1	Tr	Tr	Tr	0.1

Food No.	Food Description	Measure of edible portion	Weight (g)	Water (%)	Calories (kcal)	Protein (g)	Total fat (g)	Fatty acids: Saturated (g)	Fatty acids: Monounsaturated (g)	Fatty acids: Polyunsaturated (g)

Fruits and Fruit Juices (continued)

Food No.	Food Description	Measure of edible portion	Weight (g)	Water (%)	Calories (kcal)	Protein (g)	Total fat (g)	Saturated (g)	Monounsaturated (g)	Polyunsaturated (g)
	Strawberries									
	Raw, capped									
371	Large (1⅛" dia)	1 strawberry	18	92	5	Tr	Tr	Tr	Tr	Tr
372	Medium (1¼" dia)	1 strawberry	12	92	4	Tr	Tr	Tr	Tr	Tr
373	Sliced	1 cup	166	92	50	1	1	Tr	0.1	0.3
374	Frozen, sweetened, sliced, thawed	1 cup	255	73	245	1	Tr	Tr	Tr	0.2
	Tangerines									
375	Raw, without peel and seeds (2⅜" dia)	1 tangerine	84	88	37	1	Tr	Tr	Tr	Tr
376	Canned (mandarin oranges), light syrup, fruit and liquid	1 cup	252	83	154	1	Tr	Tr	Tr	0.1
377	Tangerine juice, canned, sweetened	1 cup	249	87	125	1	Tr	Tr	Tr	0.1
	Watermelon, raw (15" long x 7½" dia)									
378	Wedge (about 1/16 of melon)	1 wedge	286	92	92	2	1	0.1	0.3	0.4
379	Diced	1 cup	152	92	49	1	1	0.1	0.2	0.2

Grain Products

Food No.	Food Description	Measure of edible portion	Weight (g)	Water (%)	Calories (kcal)	Protein (g)	Total fat (g)	Saturated (g)	Monounsaturated (g)	Polyunsaturated (g)
	Bagels, enriched									
380	Plain	3½" bagel	71	33	195	7	1	0.2	0.1	0.5
381		4" bagel	89	33	245	9	1	0.2	0.1	0.6
382	Cinnamon raisin	3½" bagel	71	32	195	7	1	0.2	0.1	0.5
383		4" bagel	89	32	244	9	2	0.2	0.2	0.6
384	Egg	3½" bagel	71	33	197	8	1	0.3	0.3	0.5
385		4" bagel	89	33	247	9	2	0.4	0.4	0.6
386	Banana bread, prepared from recipe, with margarine	1 slice	60	29	196	3	6	1.3	2.7	1.9
	Barley, pearled									
387	Uncooked	1 cup	200	10	704	20	2	0.5	0.3	1.1
388	Cooked	1 cup	157	69	193	4	1	0.1	0.1	0.3
	Biscuits, plain or buttermilk, enriched									
389	Prepared from recipe, with 2% milk	2½" biscuit	60	29	212	4	10	2.6	4.2	2.5
390		4" biscuit	101	29	358	7	16	4.4	7.0	4.2
	Refrigerated dough, baked									
391	Regular	2½" biscuit	27	28	93	2	4	1.0	2.2	0.5
392	Lower fat	2¼" biscuit	21	28	63	2	1	0.3	0.6	0.2
	Breads, enriched									
393	Cracked wheat	1 slice	25	36	65	2	1	0.2	0.5	0.2
394	Egg bread (challah)	½" slice	40	35	115	4	2	0.6	0.9	0.4
395	French or vienna (includes sourdough)	½" slice	25	34	69	2	1	0.2	0.3	0.2
396	Indian fry (navajo) bread	5" bread	90	27	296	6	9	2.1	3.6	2.3
397		10½" bread	160	27	526	11	15	3.7	6.4	4.1
398	Italian	1 slice	20	36	54	2	1	0.2	0.2	0.3
	Mixed grain									
399	Untoasted	1 slice	26	38	65	3	1	0.2	0.4	0.2
400	Toasted	1 slice	24	32	65	3	1	0.2	0.4	0.2
	Oatmeal									
401	Untoasted	1 slice	27	37	73	2	1	0.2	0.4	0.5
402	Toasted	1 slice	25	31	73	2	1	0.2	0.4	0.5
403	Pita	4" pita	28	32	77	3	Tr	Tr	Tr	0.1
404		6½" pita	60	32	165	5	1	0.1	0.1	0.3

Food No.	Food Description	Measure of edible portion	Weight (g)	Water (%)	Calories (kcal)	Protein (g)	Total fat (g)	Fatty acids Saturated (g)	Monounsaturated (g)	Polyunsaturated (g)

Grain Products (continued)

Food No.	Food Description	Measure of edible portion	Weight (g)	Water (%)	Calories (kcal)	Protein (g)	Total fat (g)	Saturated (g)	Monounsaturated (g)	Polyunsaturated (g)
	Breads, enriched (continued)									
	Pumpernickel									
405	Untoasted	1 slice	32	38	80	3	1	0.1	0.3	0.4
406	Toasted	1 slice	29	32	80	3	1	0.1	0.3	0.4
	Raisin									
407	Untoasted	1 slice	26	34	71	2	1	0.3	0.6	0.2
408	Toasted	1 slice	24	28	71	2	1	0.3	0.6	0.2
	Rye									
409	Untoasted	1 slice	32	37	83	3	1	0.2	0.4	0.3
410	Toasted	1 slice	24	31	68	2	1	0.2	0.3	0.2
411	Rye, reduced calorie	1 slice	23	46	47	2	1	0.1	0.2	0.2
	Wheat									
412	Untoasted	1 slice	25	37	65	2	1	0.2	0.4	0.2
413	Toasted	1 slice	23	32	65	2	1	0.2	0.4	0.2
414	Wheat, reduced calorie	1 slice	23	43	46	2	1	0.1	0.1	0.2
	White									
415	Untoasted	1 slice	25	37	67	2	1	0.1	0.2	0.5
416	Toasted	1 slice	22	30	64	2	1	0.1	0.2	0.5
417	Soft crumbs	1 cup	45	37	120	4	2	0.2	0.3	0.9
418	White, reduced calorie	1 slice	23	43	48	2	1	0.1	0.2	0.1
	Bread, whole wheat									
419	Untoasted	1 slice	28	38	69	3	1	0.3	0.5	0.3
420	Toasted	1 slice	25	30	69	3	1	0.3	0.5	0.3
	Bread crumbs, dry, grated									
421	Plain, enriched	1 cup	108	6	427	14	6	1.3	2.6	1.2
422		1 oz	28	6	112	4	2	0.3	0.7	0.3
423	Seasoned, unenriched	1 cup	120	6	440	17	3	0.9	1.2	0.8
	Bread crumbs, soft. See White bread.									
424	Bread stuffing, prepared from dry mix	½ cup	100	65	178	3	9	1.7	3.8	2.6
425	Breakfast bar, cereal crust withfruit filling, fat free	1 bar	37	14	121	2	Tr	Tr	Tr	0.1
	Breakfast Cereals									
	Hot type, cooked									
	Corn (hominy) grits									
	Regular or quick, enriched									
426	White	1 cup	242	85	145	3	Tr	0.1	0.1	0.2
427	Yellow	1 cup	242	85	145	3	Tr	0.1	0.1	0.2
428	Instant, plain	1 packet	137	82	89	2	Tr	Tr	Tr	0.1
	CREAM OF WHEAT									
429	Regular	1 cup	251	87	133	4	1	0.1	0.1	0.3
430	Quick	1 cup	239	87	129	4	Tr	0.1	0.1	0.3
431	Mix'n Eat, plain	1 packet	142	82	102	3	Tr	Tr	Tr	0.2
432	MALT O MEAL	1 cup	240	88	122	4	Tr	0.1	0.1	Tr
	Oatmeal									
433	Regular, quick or instant, plain, nonfortified	1 cup	234	85	145	6	2	0.4	0.7	0.9
434	Instant, fortified, plain	1 packet	177	86	104	4	2	0.3	0.6	0.7
	QUAKER instant									
435	Apples and cinnamon	1 packet	149	79	125	3	1	0.3	0.5	0.6
436	Maple and brown sugar	1 packet	155	75	153	4	2	0.4	0.6	0.7
437	WHEATENA	1 cup	243	85	136	5	1	0.2	0.2	0.6
	Ready to eat									
438	ALL BRAN	½ cup	30	3	79	4	1	0.2	0.2	0.5
439	APPLE CINNAMON CHEERIOS	¾ cup	30	3	118	2	2	0.3	0.6	0.2
440	APPLE JACKS	1 cup	30	3	116	1	Tr	0.1	0.1	0.2

Food No.	Food Description	Measure of edible portion	Weight (g)	Water (%)	Calories (kcal)	Protein (g)	Total fat (g)	Fatty acids: Saturated (g)	Fatty acids: Monounsaturated (g)	Fatty acids: Polyunsaturated (g)

Grain Products (continued)

Food No.	Food Description	Measure of edible portion	Weight (g)	Water (%)	Calories (kcal)	Protein (g)	Total fat (g)	Saturated (g)	Monounsaturated (g)	Polyunsaturated (g)
	Breakfast Cereals (continued)									
	Ready to eat (continued)									
441	BASIC 4	1 cup	55	7	201	4	3	0.4	1.0	1.1
442	BERRY BERRY KIX	¾ cup	30	2	120	1	1	0.2	0.5	0.1
443	CAP'N CRUNCH	¾ cup	27	2	107	1	1	0.4	0.3	0.2
444	CAP'N CRUNCH'S CRUNCHBERRIES	¾ cup	26	2	104	1	1	0.3	0.3	0.2
445	CAP'N CRUNCH'S PEANUT BUTTER CRUNCH	¾ cup	27	2	112	2	2	0.5	0.8	0.5
446	CHEERIOS	1 cup	30	3	110	3	2	0.4	0.6	0.2
	CHEX									
447	Corn	1 cup	30	3	113	2	Tr	0.1	0.1	0.2
448	Honey nut	¾ cup	30	2	117	2	1	0.1	0.4	0.2
449	Multi bran	1 cup	49	3	165	4	1	0.2	0.3	0.5
450	Rice	1¼ cup	31	3	117	2	Tr	Tr	Tr	Tr
451	Wheat	1 cup	30	3	104	3	1	0.1	0.1	0.3
452	CINNAMON LIFE	1 cup	50	4	190	4	2	0.3	0.6	0.8
453	CINNAMON TOAST CRUNCH	¾ cup	30	2	124	2	3	0.5	0.9	0.5
454	COCOA KRISPIES	¾ cup	31	2	120	2	1	0.6	0.1	0.1
455	COCOA PUFFS	1 cup	30	2	119	1	1	0.2	0.3	Tr
	Corn Flakes									
456	GENERAL MILLS, TOTAL	1⅓ cup	30	3	112	2	Tr	0.2	0.1	Tr
457	KELLOGG'S	1 cup	28	3	102	2	Tr	0.1	Tr	0.1
458	CORN POPS	1 cup	31	3	118	1	Tr	0.1	0.1	Tr
459	CRISPIX	1 cup	29	3	108	2	Tr	0.1	0.1	0.1
460	Complete Wheat Bran Flakes	¾ cup	29	4	95	3	1	0.1	0.1	0.4
461	FROOT LOOPS	1 cup	30	2	117	1	1	0.4	0.2	0.3
462	FROSTED FLAKES	¾ cup	31	3	119	1	Tr	0.1	Tr	0.1
	FROSTED MINI WHEATS									
463	Regular	1 cup	51	5	173	5	1	0.2	0.1	0.6
464	Bite size	1 cup	55	5	187	5	1	0.2	0.2	0.6
465	GOLDEN GRAHAMS	¾ cup	30	3	116	2	1	0.2	0.3	0.2
466	HONEY FROSTED WHEATIES	¾ cup	30	3	110	2	Tr	0.1	Tr	Tr
467	HONEY NUT CHEERIOS	1 cup	30	2	115	3	1	0.2	0.5	0.2
468	HONEY NUT CLUSTERS	1 cup	55	3	213	5	3	0.4	1.8	0.4
469	KIX	1⅓ cup	30	2	114	2	1	0.2	0.1	Tr
470	LIFE	¾ cup	32	4	121	3	1	0.2	0.4	0.6
471	LUCKY CHARMS	1 cup	30	2	116	2	1	0.2	0.4	0.2
472	NATURE VALLEY Granola	¾ cup	55	4	248	6	10	1.3	6.5	1.9
	100% Natural Cereal									
473	With oats, honey, and raisins	½ cup	51	4	218	5	7	3.2	3.2	0.8
474	With raisins, low fat	½ cup	50	4	195	4	3	0.8	1.3	0.5
475	PRODUCT 19	1 cup	30	3	110	3	Tr	Tr	0.2	0.2
476	Puffed Rice	1 cup	14	3	56	1	Tr	Tr	Tr	Tr
477	Puffed Wheat	1 cup	12	3	44	2	Tr	Tr	Tr	Tr
	Raisin Bran									
478	GENERAL MILLS, TOTAL	1 cup	55	9	178	4	1	0.2	0.2	0.2
479	KELLOGG'S	1 cup	61	8	186	6	1	0.0	0.2	0.8
480	RAISIN NUT BRAN	1 cup	55	5	209	5	4	0.7	1.9	0.5
481	REESE'S PEANUT BUTTER PUFFS	¾ cup	30	2	129	3	3	0.6	1.4	0.6
482	RICE KRISPIES	1¼ cup	33	3	124	2	Tr	0.1	0.1	0.2

Grain Products (continued)

Food No.	Food Description	Measure of edible portion	Weight (g)	Water (%)	Calories (kcal)	Protein (g)	Total fat (g)	Fatty acids Saturated (g)	Mono-unsaturated (g)	Poly-unsaturated (g)
	Breakfast Cereals (continued)									
	Ready to eat (continued)									
483	RICE KRISPIES TREATS cereal	¾ cup	30	4	120	1	2	0.4	1.0	0.2
484	SHREDDED WHEAT	2 biscuits	46	4	156	5	1	0.1	NA	NA
485	SMACKS	¾ cup	27	3	103	2	1	0.3	0.1	0.2
486	SPECIAL K	1 cup	31	3	115	6	Tr	0.0	0.0	0.2
487	QUAKER Toasted Oatmeal, Honey Nut	1 cup	49	3	191	5	3	0.5	1.2	0.7
488	TOTAL, Whole Grain	¾ cup	30	3	105	3	1	0.2	0.1	0.1
489	TRIX	1 cup	30	2	122	1	2	0.4	0.9	0.3
490	WHEATIES	1 cup	30	3	110	3	1	0.2	0.2	0.2
	Brownies, without icing									
	Commercially prepared									
491	Regular, large (2¾" sq x ⅞")	1 brownie	56	14	227	3	9	2.4	5.0	1.3
492	Fat free, 2" sq	1 brownie	28	12	89	1	Tr	0.2	0.1	Tr
493	Prepared from dry mix, reduced calorie, 2" sq	1 brownie	22	13	84	1	2	1.1	1.0	0.2
494	Buckwheat flour, whole groat	1 cup	120	11	402	15	4	0.8	1.1	1.1
495	Buckwheat groats, roasted (kasha), cooked	1 cup	168	76	155	6	1	0.2	0.3	0.3
	Bulgur									
496	Uncooked	1 cup	140	9	479	17	2	0.3	0.2	0.8
497	Cooked	1 cup	182	78	151	6	Tr	0.1	0.1	0.2
	Cakes, prepared from dry mix									
498	Angelfood (1/12 of 10" dia)	1 piece	50	33	129	3	Tr	Tr	Tr	0.1
499	Yellow, light, with water, egg whites, no frosting (1/12 of 9" dia)	1 piece	69	37	181	3	2	1.1	0.9	0.2
	Cakes, prepared from recipe									
500	Chocolate, without frosting (1/12 of 9" dia)	1 piece	95	24	340	5	14	5.2	5.7	2.6
501	Gingerbread (1/9 of 8" square)	1 piece	74	28	263	3	12	3.1	5.3	3.1
502	Pineapple upside down (1/9 of 8" square)	1 piece	115	32	367	4	14	3.4	6.0	3.8
503	Shortcake, biscuit type (about 3" dia)	1 shortcake	65	28	225	4	9	2.5	3.9	2.4
504	Sponge (1/12 of 16-oz cake)	1 piece	63	29	187	5	3	0.8	1.0	0.4
	White									
505	With coconut frosting (1/12 of 9" dia)	1 piece	112	21	399	5	12	4.4	4.1	2.4
506	Without frosting (1/12 of 9" dia)	1 piece	74	23	264	4	9	2.4	3.9	2.3
	Cakes, commercially prepared									
507	Angelfood (1/12 of 12-oz cake)	1 piece	28	33	72	2	Tr	Tr	Tr	0.1
508	Boston cream (1/6 of pie)	1 piece	92	45	232	2	8	2.2	4.2	0.9
509	Chocolate with chocolate frosting (1/8 of 18-oz cake)	1 piece	64	23	235	3	10	3.1	5.6	1.2
510	Coffeecake, crumb (1/9 of 20-oz cake)	1 piece	63	22	263	4	15	3.7	8.2	2.0
511	Fruitcake	1 piece	43	25	139	1	4	0.5	1.8	1.4
	Pound									
512	Butter (1/12 of 12-oz cake)	1 piece	28	25	109	2	6	3.2	1.7	0.3
513	Fat free (3¼" x 2¾" x ⅝" slice)	1 slice	28	31	79	2	Tr	0.1	Tr	0.1

Food No.	Food Description	Measure of edible portion	Weight (g)	Water (%)	Calories (kcal)	Protein (g)	Total fat (g)	Fatty acids Saturated (g)	Fatty acids Monounsaturated (g)	Fatty acids Polyunsaturated (g)

Grain Products (continued)

Food No.	Food Description	Measure of edible portion	Weight (g)	Water (%)	Calories (kcal)	Protein (g)	Total fat (g)	Saturated (g)	Monounsaturated (g)	Polyunsaturated (g)
	Cakes, commercially prepared (continued)									
	Snack cakes									
514	Chocolate, creme filled, with frosting	1 cupcake	50	20	188	2	7	1.4	2.8	2.6
515	Chocolate, with frosting, low fat	1 cupcake	43	23	131	2	2	0.5	0.8	0.2
516	Sponge, creme filled	1 cake	43	20	155	1	5	1.1	1.7	1.4
517	Sponge, individual shortcake	1 shortcake	30	30	87	2	1	0.2	0.3	0.1
	Yellow									
518	With chocolate frosting	1 piece	64	22	243	2	11	3.0	6.1	1.4
519	With vanilla frosting	1 piece	64	22	239	2	9	1.5	3.9	3.3
520	Cheesecake (⅙ of 17-oz cake)	1 piece	80	46	257	4	18	7.9	6.9	1.3
521	Cheese flavor puffs or twists	1 oz	28	2	157	2	10	1.9	5.7	1.3
522	CHEX mix	1 oz (about ⅔ cup)	28	4	120	3	5	1.6	NA	NA
	Cookies									
523	Butter, commercially prepared	1 cookie	5	5	23	Tr	1	0.6	0.3	Tr
	Chocolate chip, medium (2¼"-2½" dia)									
	Commercially prepared									
524	Regular	1 cookie	10	4	48	1	2	0.7	1.2	0.2
525	Reduced fat	1 cookie	10	4	45	1	2	0.4	0.6	0.5
526	From refrigerated dough (spooned from roll)	1 cookie	26	3	128	1	6	2.0	2.9	0.6
527	Prepared from recipe, with margarine	1 cookie	16	6	78	1	5	1.3	1.7	1.3
528	Devil's food, commercially prepared, fat free	1 cookie	16	18	49	1	Tr	0.1	Tr	Tr
529	Fig bar	1 cookie	16	17	56	1	1	0.2	0.5	0.4
	Molasses									
530	Medium	1 cookie	15	6	65	1	2	0.5	1.1	0.3
531	Large (3½"-4" dia)	1 cookie	32	6	138	2	4	1.0	2.3	0.6
	Oatmeal									
	Commercially prepared, with or without raisins									
532	Regular, large	1 cookie	25	6	113	2	5	1.1	2.5	0.6
533	Soft type	1 cookie	15	11	61	1	2	0.5	1.2	0.3
534	Fat free	1 cookie	11	13	36	1	Tr	Tr	Tr	0.1
535	Prepared from recipe, with raisins (2⅝" dia)	1 cookie	15	6	65	1	2	0.5	1.0	0.8
	Peanut butter									
536	Commercially prepared	1 cookie	15	6	72	1	4	0.7	1.9	0.8
537	Prepared from recipe, with margarine (3" dia)	1 cookie	20	6	95	2	5	0.9	2.2	1.4
	Sandwich type, with creme filling									
538	Chocolate cookie	1 cookie	10	2	47	Tr	2	0.4	0.9	0.7
	Vanilla cookie									
539	Oval	1 cookie	15	2	72	1	3	0.4	1.3	1.1
540	Round	1 cookie	10	2	48	Tr	2	0.3	0.8	0.8
	Shortbread, commercially prepared									
541	Plain (1⅝" sq)	1 cookie	8	4	40	Tr	2	0.5	1.1	0.3
	Pecan									
542	Regular (2" dia)	1 cookie	14	3	76	1	5	1.1	2.6	0.6
543	Reduced fat	1 cookie	16	5	73	1	3	0.6	1.6	0.4

Table 9. Nutritive Value of the Edible Part of Food

Grain Products (continued)

Food No.	Food Description	Measure of edible portion	Weight (g)	Water (%)	Calories (kcal)	Protein (g)	Total fat (g)	Fatty acids: Saturated (g)	Fatty acids: Monounsaturated (g)	Fatty acids: Polyunsaturated (g)
	Cookies (continued)									
	Sugar									
544	Commercially prepared	1 cookie	15	5	72	1	3	0.8	1.8	0.4
545	From refrigerated dough	1 cookie	15	5	73	1	3	0.9	2.0	0.4
546	Prepared from recipe, with margarine (3" dia)	1 cookie	14	9	66	1	3	0.7	1.4	1.0
547	Vanilla wafer, lower fat, medium size	1 cookie	4	5	18	Tr	1	0.2	0.3	0.2
	Corn chips									
548	Plain	1 oz	28	1	153	2	9	1.3	2.7	4.7
549	Barbecue flavor	1 oz	28	1	148	2	9	1.3	2.7	4.6
	Cornbread									
550	Prepared from mix, piece 3¾" x 2½" x ¾"	1 piece	60	32	188	4	6	1.6	3.1	0.7
551	Prepared from recipe, with 2% milk, piece 2½" sq x 1½"	1 piece	65	39	173	4	5	1.0	1.2	2.1
	Cornmeal, yellow, dry form									
552	Whole grain	1 cup	122	10	442	10	4	0.6	1.2	2.0
553	Degermed, enriched	1 cup	138	12	505	12	2	0.3	0.6	1.0
554	Self rising, degermed, enriched	1 cup	138	10	490	12	2	0.3	0.6	1.0
555	Cornstarch	1 tbsp	8	8	30	Tr	Tr	Tr	Tr	Tr
	Couscous									
556	Uncooked	1 cup	173	9	650	22	1	0.2	0.2	0.4
557	Cooked	1 cup	157	73	176	6	Tr	Tr	Tr	0.1
	Crackers									
558	Cheese, 1" sq	10 crackers	10	3	50	1	3	0.9	1.2	0.2
	Graham, plain									
559	2½" sq	2 squares	14	4	59	1	1	0.2	0.6	0.5
560	Crushed	1 cup	84	4	355	6	8	1.3	3.4	3.2
561	Melba toast, plain	4 pieces	20	5	78	2	1	0.1	0.2	0.3
562	Rye wafer, whole grain, plain	1 wafer	11	5	37	1	Tr	Tr	Tr	Tr
	Saltine									
563	Square	4 crackers	12	4	52	1	1	0.4	0.8	0.2
564	Oyster type	1 cup	45	4	195	4	5	1.3	2.9	0.8
	Sandwich type									
565	Wheat with cheese	1 sandwich	7	4	33	1	1	0.4	0.8	0.2
566	Cheese with peanut butter	1 sandwich	7	4	34	1	2	0.4	0.8	0.3
	Standard snack type									
567	Bite size	1 cup	62	4	311	5	16	2.3	6.6	5.9
568	Round	4 crackers	12	4	60	1	3	0.5	1.3	1.1
569	Wheat, thin square	4 crackers	8	3	38	1	2	0.4	0.9	0.2
570	Whole wheat	4 crackers	16	3	71	1	3	0.5	0.9	1.1
571	Croissant, butter	1 croissant	57	23	231	5	12	6.6	3.1	0.6
572	Croutons, seasoned	1 cup	40	4	186	4	7	2.1	3.8	0.9
	Danish pastry, enriched									
573	Cheese filled	1 danish	71	31	266	6	16	4.8	8.0	1.8
574	Fruit filled	1 danish	71	27	263	4	13	3.5	7.1	1.7
	Doughnuts									
575	Cake type	1 hole	14	21	59	1	3	0.5	1.3	1.1
576		1 medium	47	21	198	2	11	1.7	4.4	3.7
577	Yeast leavened, glazed	1 hole	13	25	52	1	3	0.8	1.7	0.4
578		1 medium	60	25	242	4	14	3.5	7.7	1.7
579	Eclair, prepared from recipe, 5" x 2" x 1¾"	1 eclair	100	52	262	6	16	4.1	6.5	3.9
	English muffin, plain, enriched									
580	Untoasted	1 muffin	57	42	134	4	1	0.1	0.2	0.5
581	Toasted	1 muffin	52	37	133	4	1	0.1	0.2	0.5

Food No.	Food Description	Measure of edible portion	Weight (g)	Water (%)	Calories (kcal)	Protein (g)	Total fat (g)	Fatty acids: Saturated (g)	Fatty acids: Monounsaturated (g)	Fatty acids: Polyunsaturated (g)

Grain Products (continued)

Food No.	Food Description	Measure of edible portion	Weight (g)	Water (%)	Calories (kcal)	Protein (g)	Total fat (g)	Saturated (g)	Monounsaturated (g)	Polyunsaturated (g)
	French toast									
582	Prepared from recipe, with 2% milk, fried in margarine	1 slice	65	55	149	5	7	1.8	2.9	1.7
583	Frozen, ready to heat	1 slice	59	53	126	4	4	0.9	1.2	0.7
	Granola bar									
584	Hard, plain	1 bar	28	4	134	3	6	0.7	1.2	3.4
	Soft, uncoated									
585	Chocolate chip	1 bar	28	5	119	2	5	2.9	1.0	0.6
586	Raisin	1 bar	28	6	127	2	5	2.7	0.8	0.9
587	Soft, chocolate-coated, peanut butter	1 bar	28	3	144	3	9	4.8	1.9	0.5
588	Macaroni (elbows), enriched, cooked	1 cup	140	66	197	7	1	0.1	0.1	0.4
589	Matzo, plain	1 matzo	28	4	112	3	Tr	0.1	Tr	0.2
	Muffins									
	Blueberry									
590	Commercially prepared (2¾" dia x 2")	1 muffin	57	38	158	3	4	0.8	1.1	1.4
591	Prepared from mix (2¼" dia x 1¾")	1 muffin	50	36	150	3	4	0.7	1.8	1.5
592	Prepared from recipe, with 2% milk	1 muffin	57	40	162	4	6	1.2	1.5	3.1
593	Bran with raisins, toaster type, toasted	1 muffin	34	27	106	2	3	0.5	0.8	1.7
	Corn									
594	Commercially prepared (2½" dia x 2¼")	1 muffin	57	33	174	3	5	0.8	1.2	1.8
595	Prepared from mix (2¼" dia x 1½")	1 muffin	50	31	161	4	5	1.4	2.6	0.6
596	Oat bran, commercially prepared (2½" dia x 2¼")	1 muffin	57	35	154	4	4	0.6	1.0	2.4
597	Noodles, chow mein, canned	1 cup	45	1	237	4	14	2.0	3.5	7.8
	Noodles (egg noodles), enriched, cooked									
598	Regular	1 cup	160	69	213	8	2	0.5	0.7	0.7
599	Spinach	1 cup	160	69	211	8	3	0.6	0.8	0.6
600	NUTRI GRAIN Cereal Bar, fruit filled	1 bar	37	15	136	2	3	0.6	1.9	0.3
	Oat bran									
601	Uncooked	1 cup	94	7	231	16	7	1.2	2.2	2.6
602	Cooked	1 cup	219	84	88	7	2	0.4	0.6	0.7
603	Oriental snack mix	1 oz (about ¼ cup)	28	3	156	5	7	1.1	2.8	3.0
	Pancakes, plain (4" dia)									
604	Frozen, ready to heat	1 pancake	36	45	82	2	1	0.3	0.4	0.3
605	Prepared from complete mix	1 pancake	38	53	74	2	1	0.2	0.3	0.3
606	Prepared from incomplete mix, with 2% milk, egg and oil	1 pancake	38	53	83	3	3	0.8	0.8	1.1
	Pie crust, baked									
	Standard type									
607	From recipe	1 pie shell	180	10	949	12	62	15.5	27.3	16.4
608	From frozen	1 pie shell	126	11	648	6	41	13.3	19.8	5.1
609	Graham cracker	1 pie shell	239	4	1,181	10	60	12.4	27.2	16.5

Food No.	Food Description	Measure of edible portion	Weight (g)	Water (%)	Calories (kcal)	Protein (g)	Total fat (g)	Fatty acids: Saturated (g)	Fatty acids: Monounsaturated (g)	Fatty acids: Polyunsaturated (g)

Grain Products (continued)

Food No.	Food Description	Measure of edible portion	Weight (g)	Water (%)	Calories (kcal)	Protein (g)	Total fat (g)	Saturated (g)	Monounsaturated (g)	Polyunsaturated (g)
	Pies									
	Commercially prepared (⅙ of 8" dia)									
610	Apple	1 piece	117	52	277	2	13	4.4	5.1	2.6
611	Blueberry	1 piece	117	53	271	2	12	2.0	5.0	4.1
612	Cherry	1 piece	117	46	304	2	13	3.0	6.8	2.4
613	Chocolate creme	1 piece	113	44	344	3	22	5.6	12.6	2.7
614	Coconut custard	1 piece	104	49	270	6	14	6.1	5.7	1.2
615	Lemon meringue	1 piece	113	42	303	2	10	2.0	3.0	4.1
616	Pecan	1 piece	113	19	452	5	21	4.0	12.1	3.6
617	Pumpkin	1 piece	109	58	229	4	10	1.9	4.4	3.4
	Prepared from recipe (⅛ of 9" dia)									
618	Apple	1 piece	155	47	411	4	19	4.7	8.4	5.2
619	Blueberry	1 piece	147	51	360	4	17	4.3	7.5	4.5
620	Cherry	1 piece	180	46	486	5	22	5.4	9.6	5.8
621	Lemon meringue	1 piece	127	43	362	5	16	4.0	7.1	4.2
622	Pecan	1 piece	122	20	503	6	27	4.9	13.6	7.0
623	Pumpkin	1 piece	155	59	316	7	14	4.9	5.7	2.8
624	Fried, cherry	1 pie	128	38	404	4	21	3.1	9.5	6.9
	Popcorn									
625	Air popped, unsalted	1 cup	8	4	31	1	Tr	Tr	0.1	0.2
626	Oil popped, salted	1 cup	11	3	55	1	3	0.5	0.9	1.5
	Caramel coated									
627	With peanuts	1 cup	42	3	168	3	3	0.4	1.1	1.4
628	Without peanuts	1 cup	35	3	152	1	5	1.3	1.0	1.6
629	Cheese flavor	1 cup	11	3	58	1	4	0.7	1.1	1.7
630	Popcorn cake	1 cake	10	5	38	1	Tr	Tr	0.1	0.1
	Pretzels, made with enriched flour									
631	Stick, 2¼" long	10 pretzels	3	3	11	Tr	Tr	Tr	Tr	Tr
632	Twisted, regular	10 pretzels	60	3	229	5	2	0.5	0.8	0.7
633	Twisted, dutch, 2¾" x 2⅝"	1 pretzel	16	3	61	1	1	0.1	0.2	0.2
	Rice									
634	Brown, long grain, cooked	1 cup	195	73	216	5	2	0.4	0.6	0.6
	White, long grain, enriched									
	Regular									
635	Raw	1 cup	185	12	675	13	1	0.3	0.4	0.3
636	Cooked	1 cup	158	68	205	4	Tr	0.1	0.1	0.1
637	Instant, prepared	1 cup	165	76	162	3	Tr	0.1	0.1	0.1
	Parboiled									
638	Raw	1 cup	185	10	686	13	1	0.3	0.3	0.3
639	Cooked	1 cup	175	72	200	4	Tr	0.1	0.1	0.1
640	Wild, cooked	1 cup	164	74	166	7	1	0.1	0.1	0.3
641	Rice cake, brown rice, plain	1 cake	9	6	35	1	Tr	0.1	0.1	0.1
642	RICE KRISPIES Treat Squares	1 bar	22	6	91	1	2	0.3	0.6	1.1
	Rolls									
643	Dinner	1 roll	28	32	84	2	2	0.5	1.0	0.3
644	Hamburger or hotdog	1 roll	43	34	123	4	2	0.5	0.4	1.1
645	Hard, kaiser	1 roll	57	31	167	6	2	0.3	0.6	1.0
	Spaghetti, cooked									
646	Enriched	1 cup	140	66	197	7	1	0.1	0.1	0.4
647	Whole wheat	1 cup	140	67	174	7	1	0.1	0.1	0.3
	Sweet rolls, cinnamon									
648	Commercial, with raisins	1 roll	60	25	223	4	10	1.8	2.9	4.5
649	Refrigerated dough, baked, with frosting	1 roll	30	23	109	2	4	1.0	2.2	0.5

Table 9. Nutritive Value of the Edible Part of Food

Food No.	Food Description	Measure of edible portion	Weight (g)	Water (%)	Calories (kcal)	Protein (g)	Total fat (g)	Fatty acids: Saturated (g)	Fatty acids: Monounsaturated (g)	Fatty acids: Polyunsaturated (g)
	Grain Products (continued)									
650	Taco shell, baked	1 medium	13	6	62	1	3	0.4	1.2	1.1
651	Tapioca, pearl, dry	1 cup	152	11	544	Tr	Tr	Tr	Tr	Tr
	Toaster pastries									
652	Brown sugar cinnamon	1 pastry	50	11	206	3	7	1.8	4.0	0.9
653	Chocolate with frosting	1 pastry	52	13	201	3	5	1.0	2.7	1.1
654	Fruit filled	1 pastry	52	12	204	2	5	0.8	2.2	2.0
655	Low fat	1 pastry	52	12	193	2	3	0.7	1.7	0.5
	Tortilla chips									
	Plain									
656	Regular	1 oz	28	2	142	2	7	1.4	4.4	1.0
657	Low fat, baked	10 chips	14	2	54	2	1	0.1	0.2	0.4
	Nacho flavor									
658	Regular	1 oz	28	2	141	2	7	1.4	4.3	1.0
659	Light, reduced fat	1 oz	28	1	126	2	4	0.8	2.5	0.6
	Tortillas, ready to cook (about 6" dia)									
660	Corn	1 tortilla	26	44	58	1	1	0.1	0.2	0.3
661	Flour	1 tortilla	32	27	104	3	2	0.6	1.2	0.3
	Waffles, plain									
662	Prepared from recipe, 7" dia	1 waffle	75	42	218	6	11	2.1	2.6	5.1
663	Frozen, toasted, 4" dia	1 waffle	33	42	87	2	3	0.5	1.1	0.9
664	Low fat, 4" dia	1 waffle	35	43	83	2	1	0.3	0.4	0.4
	Wheat flours									
	All purpose, enriched									
665	Sifted, spooned	1 cup	115	12	419	12	1	0.2	0.1	0.5
666	Unsifted, spooned	1 cup	125	12	455	13	1	0.2	0.1	0.5
667	Bread, enriched	1 cup	137	13	495	16	2	0.3	0.2	1.0
668	Cake or pastry flour, enriched, unsifted, spooned	1 cup	137	13	496	11	1	0.2	0.1	0.5
669	Self rising, enriched, unsifted, spooned	1 cup	125	11	443	12	1	0.2	0.1	0.5
670	Whole wheat, from hard wheats, stirred, spooned	1 cup	120	10	407	16	2	0.4	0.3	0.9
671	Wheat germ, toasted, plain	1 tbsp	7	6	27	2	1	0.1	0.1	0.5
	Legumes, Nuts, and Seeds									
	Almonds, shelled									
672	Sliced	1 cup	95	5	549	20	48	3.7	30.5	11.6
673	Whole	1 oz (24 nuts)	28	5	164	6	14	1.1	9.1	3.5
	Beans, dry									
	Cooked									
674	Black	1 cup	172	66	227	15	1	0.2	0.1	0.4
675	Great Northern	1 cup	177	69	209	15	1	0.2	Tr	0.3
676	Kidney, red	1 cup	177	67	225	15	1	0.1	0.1	0.5
677	Lima, large	1 cup	188	70	216	15	1	0.2	0.1	0.3
678	Pea (navy)	1 cup	182	63	258	16	1	0.3	0.1	0.4
679	Pinto	1 cup	171	64	234	14	1	0.2	0.2	0.3
	Canned, solids and liquid									
	Baked beans									
680	Plain or vegetarian	1 cup	254	73	236	12	1	0.3	0.1	0.5
681	With frankfurters	1 cup	259	69	368	17	17	6.1	7.3	2.2
682	With pork in tomato sauce	1 cup	253	73	248	13	3	1.0	1.1	0.3
683	With pork in sweet sauce	1 cup	253	71	281	13	4	1.4	1.6	0.5
684	Kidney, red	1 cup	256	77	218	13	1	0.1	0.1	0.5
685	Lima, large	1 cup	241	77	190	12	Tr	0.1	Tr	0.2
686	White	1 cup	262	70	307	19	1	0.2	0.1	0.3

Table 9. Nutritive Value of the Edible Part of Food

Legumes, Nuts, and Seeds (continued)

Food No.	Food Description	Measure of edible portion	Weight (g)	Water (%)	Calories (kcal)	Protein (g)	Total fat (g)	Fatty acids: Saturated (g)	Fatty acids: Monounsaturated (g)	Fatty acids: Polyunsaturated (g)
	Black eyed peas, dry									
687	Cooked	1 cup	172	70	200	13	1	0.2	0.1	0.4
688	Canned, solids and liquid	1 cup	240	80	185	11	1	0.3	0.1	0.6
689	Brazil nuts, shelled	1 oz (6-8 nuts)	28	3	186	4	19	4.6	6.5	6.8
690	Carob flour	1 cup	103	4	229	5	1	0.1	0.2	0.2
	Cashews, salted									
691	Dry roasted	1 oz	28	2	163	4	13	2.6	7.7	2.2
692	Oil roasted	1 cup	130	4	749	21	63	12.4	36.9	10.6
693		1 oz (18 nuts)	28	4	163	5	14	2.7	8.1	2.3
694	Chestnuts, European, roasted, shelled	1 cup	143	40	350	5	3	0.6	1.1	1.2
	Chickpeas, dry									
695	Cooked	1 cup	164	60	269	15	4	0.4	1.0	1.9
696	Canned, solids and liquid	1 cup	240	70	286	12	3	0.3	0.6	1.2
	Coconut									
	Raw									
697	Piece, about 2" x 2" x ½"	1 piece	45	47	159	1	15	13.4	0.6	0.2
698	Shredded, not packed	1 cup	80	47	283	3	27	23.8	1.1	0.3
699	Dried, sweetened, shredded	1 cup	93	13	466	3	33	29.3	1.4	0.4
700	Hazelnuts (filberts), chopped	1 cup	115	5	722	17	70	5.1	52.5	9.1
701		1 oz	28	5	178	4	17	1.3	12.9	2.2
702	Hummus, commercial	1 tbsp	14	67	23	1	1	0.2	0.6	0.5
703	Lentils, dry, cooked	1 cup	198	70	230	18	1	0.1	0.1	0.3
704	Macadamia nuts, dry roasted, salted	1 cup	134	2	959	10	102	16.0	79.4	2.0
705		1 oz (10-12 nuts)	28	2	203	2	22	3.4	16.8	0.4
	Mixed nuts, with peanuts, salted									
706	Dry roasted	1 oz	28	2	168	5	15	2.0	8.9	3.1
707	Oil roasted	1 oz	28	2	175	5	16	2.5	9.0	3.8
	Peanuts									
	Dry roasted									
708	Salted	1 oz (about 28)	28	2	166	7	14	2.0	7.0	4.4
709	Unsalted	1 cup	146	2	854	35	73	10.1	36.0	22.9
710		1 oz (about 28)	28	2	166	7	14	2.0	7.0	4.4
711	Oil roasted, salted	1 cup	144	2	837	38	71	9.9	35.2	22.4
712		1 oz	28	2	165	7	14	1.9	6.9	4.4
	Peanut butter									
	Regular									
713	Smooth style	1 tbsp	16	1	95	4	8	1.7	3.9	2.2
714	Chunk style	1 tbsp	16	1	94	4	8	1.5	3.8	2.3
715	Reduced fat, smooth	1 tbsp	18	1	94	5	6	1.3	2.9	1.8
716	Peas, split, dry, cooked	1 cup	196	69	231	16	1	0.1	0.2	0.3
717	Pecans, halves	1 cup	108	4	746	10	78	6.7	44.0	23.3
718		1 oz (20 halves)	28	4	196	3	20	1.8	11.6	6.1
719	Pine nuts (pignolia), shelled	1 oz	28	7	160	7	14	2.2	5.4	6.1
720		1 tbsp	9	7	49	2	4	0.7	1.6	1.8
721	Pistachio nuts, dry roasted, with salt, shelled	1 oz (47 nuts)	28	2	161	6	13	1.6	6.8	3.9
722	Pumpkin and squash kernels, roasted, with salt	1 oz (142 seeds)	28	7	148	9	12	2.3	3.7	5.4
723	Refried beans, canned	1 cup	252	76	237	14	3	1.2	1.4	0.4
724	Sesame seeds	1 tbsp	8	5	47	2	4	0.6	1.7	1.9
725	Soybeans, dry, cooked	1 cup	172	63	298	29	15	2.2	3.4	8.7
	Soy products									
726	Miso	1 cup	275	41	567	32	17	2.4	3.7	9.4
727	Soy milk	1 cup	245	93	81	7	5	0.5	0.8	2.0

Food No.	Food Description	Measure of edible portion	Weight (g)	Water (%)	Calories (kcal)	Protein (g)	Total fat (g)	Fatty acids Saturated (g)	Fatty acids Monounsaturated (g)	Fatty acids Polyunsaturated (g)

Legumes, Nuts, and Seeds (continued)

Food No.	Food Description	Measure of edible portion	Weight (g)	Water (%)	Calories (kcal)	Protein (g)	Total fat (g)	Saturated (g)	Monounsaturated (g)	Polyunsaturated (g)
	Soy products (continued)									
	Tofu									
728	Firm	¼ block	81	84	62	7	4	0.5	0.8	2.0
729	Soft, piece 2½" x 2¾" x 1"	1 piece	120	87	73	8	4	0.6	1.0	2.5
730	Sunflower seed kernels, dry roasted, with salt	¼ cup	32	1	186	6	16	1.7	3.0	10.5
731		1 oz	28	1	165	5	14	1.5	2.7	9.3
732	Tahini	1 tbsp	15	3	89	3	8	1.1	3.0	3.5
733	Walnuts, English	1 cup, chopped	120	4	785	18	78	7.4	10.7	56.6
734		1 oz (14 halves)	28	4	185	4	18	1.7	2.5	13.4

Meat and Meat Products

Food No.	Food Description	Measure of edible portion	Weight (g)	Water (%)	Calories (kcal)	Protein (g)	Total fat (g)	Saturated (g)	Monounsaturated (g)	Polyunsaturated (g)
	Beef, cooked									
	Cuts braised, simmered, or pot roasted									
	Relatively fat, such as chuck blade, piece, 2½" x 2½" x ¾"									
735	Lean and fat	3 oz	85	47	293	23	22	8.7	9.4	0.8
736	Lean only	3 oz	85	55	213	26	11	4.3	4.8	0.4
	Relatively lean, such as bottom round, piece, 4⅛" x 2¼" x ½"									
737	Lean and fat	3 oz	85	52	234	24	14	5.4	6.2	0.5
738	Lean only	3 oz	85	58	178	27	7	2.4	3.1	0.3
	Ground beef, broiled									
739	83% lean	3 oz	85	57	218	22	14	5.5	6.1	0.5
740	79% lean	3 oz	85	56	231	21	16	6.2	6.9	0.6
741	73% lean	3 oz	85	54	246	20	18	6.9	7.7	0.7
742	Liver, fried, slice, 6½" x 2⅜" x ⅜"	3 oz	85	56	184	23	7	2.3	1.4	1.5
	Roast, oven cooked, no liquid added									
	Relatively fat, such as rib, 2 pieces, 4⅛" x 2¼" x ¼"									
743	Lean and fat	3 oz	85	47	304	19	25	9.9	10.6	0.9
744	Lean only	3 oz	85	59	195	23	11	4.2	4.5	0.3
	Relatively lean, such as eye of round, 2 pieces, 2½" x 2½" x ⅜"									
745	Lean and fat	3 oz	85	59	195	23	11	4.2	4.7	0.4
746	Lean only	3 oz	85	65	143	25	4	1.5	1.8	0.1
	Steak, sirloin, broiled, piece, 2½" x 2½" x ¾"									
747	Lean and fat	3 oz	85	57	219	24	13	5.2	5.6	0.5
748	Lean only	3 oz	85	62	166	26	6	2.4	2.6	0.2
749	Beef, canned, corned	3 oz	85	58	213	23	13	5.3	5.1	0.5
750	Beef, dried, chipped	1 oz	28	57	47	8	1	0.5	0.5	0.1
	Lamb, cooked									
	Chops									
	Arm, braised									
751	Lean and fat	3 oz	85	44	294	26	20	8.4	8.7	1.5
752	Lean only	3 oz	85	49	237	30	12	4.3	5.2	0.8
	Loin, broiled									
753	Lean and fat	3 oz	85	52	269	21	20	8.4	8.2	1.4
754	Lean only	3 oz	85	61	184	25	8	3.0	3.6	0.5

Food No.	Food Description	Measure of edible portion	Weight (g)	Water (%)	Calories (kcal)	Protein (g)	Total fat (g)	Fatty acids Saturated (g)	Monounsaturated (g)	Polyunsaturated (g)

Meat and Meat Products (continued)

Food No.	Food Description	Measure of edible portion	Weight (g)	Water (%)	Calories (kcal)	Protein (g)	Total fat (g)	Saturated (g)	Monounsaturated (g)	Polyunsaturated (g)
	Lamb (continued)									
	Leg, roasted, 2 pieces, 4⅛" x 2¼" x ¼"									
755	Lean and fat	3 oz	85	57	219	22	14	5.9	5.9	1.0
756	Lean only	3 oz	85	64	162	24	7	2.3	2.9	0.4
	Rib, roasted, 3 pieces, 2½" x 2½" x ¼"									
757	Lean and fat	3 oz	85	48	305	18	25	10.9	10.6	1.8
758	Lean only	3 oz	85	60	197	22	11	4.0	5.0	0.7
	Pork, cured, cooked									
	Bacon									
759	Regular	3 medium slices	19	13	109	6	9	3.3	4.5	1.1
760	Canadian style (6 slices per 6-oz pkg)	2 slices	47	62	86	11	4	1.3	1.9	0.4
	Ham, light cure, roasted, 2 pieces, 4⅛" x 2¼" x ¼"									
761	Lean and fat	3 oz	85	58	207	18	14	5.1	6.7	1.5
762	Lean only	3 oz	85	66	133	21	5	1.6	2.2	0.5
763	Ham, canned, roasted, 2 pieces, 4⅛" x 2¼" x ¼"	3 oz	85	67	142	18	7	2.4	3.5	0.8
	Pork, fresh, cooked									
	Chop, loin (cut 3 per lb with bone)									
	Broiled									
764	Lean and fat	3 oz	85	58	204	24	11	4.1	5.0	0.8
765	Lean only	3 oz	85	61	172	26	7	2.5	3.1	0.5
	Pan fried									
766	Lean and fat	3 oz	85	53	235	25	14	5.1	6.0	1.6
767	Lean only	3 oz	85	57	197	27	9	3.1	3.8	1.1
	Ham (leg), roasted, piece, 2½" x 2½" x ¾"									
768	Lean and fat	3 oz	85	55	232	23	15	5.5	6.7	1.4
769	Lean only	3 oz	85	61	179	25	8	2.8	3.8	0.7
	Rib roast, piece, 2½" x 2½" x ¾"									
770	Lean and fat	3 oz	85	56	217	23	13	5.0	5.9	1.1
771	Lean only	3 oz	85	59	190	24	9	3.7	4.5	0.7
	Ribs, lean and fat, cooked									
772	Backribs, roasted	3 oz	85	45	315	21	25	9.3	11.4	2.0
773	Country style, braised	3 oz	85	54	252	20	18	6.8	7.9	1.6
774	Spareribs, braised	3 oz	85	40	337	25	26	9.5	11.5	2.3
	Shoulder cut, braised, 3 pieces, 2½" x 2½" x ¼"									
775	Lean and fat	3 oz	85	48	280	24	20	7.2	8.8	1.9
776	Lean only	3 oz	85	54	211	27	10	3.5	4.9	1.0
	Sausages and luncheon meats									
777	Bologna, beef and pork (8 slices per 8-oz pkg)	2 slices	57	54	180	7	16	6.1	7.6	1.4
778	Braunschweiger (6 slices per 6-oz pkg)	2 slices	57	48	205	8	18	6.2	8.5	2.1
779	Brown and serve, cooked, link, 4" x ⅞" raw	2 links	26	45	103	4	9	3.4	4.5	1.0
	Canned, minced luncheon meat									
780	Pork, ham, and chicken, reduced sodium (7 slices per 7-oz can)	2 slices	57	56	172	7	15	5.1	7.1	1.5
781	Pork with ham (12 slices per 12-oz can)	2 slices	57	52	188	8	17	5.7	7.7	1.2
782	Pork and chicken (12 slices per 12-oz can)	2 slices	57	64	117	9	8	2.7	3.8	0.8

Food No.	Food Description	Measure of edible portion	Weight (g)	Water (%)	Calories (kcal)	Protein (g)	Total fat (g)	Fatty acids: Saturated (g)	Fatty acids: Monounsaturated (g)	Fatty acids: Polyunsaturated (g)
	Meat and Meat Products (continued)									
	Sausages and luncheon meats (continued)									
783	Chopped ham (8 slices per 6-oz pkg)	2 slices	21	64	48	4	4	1.2	1.7	0.4
	Cooked ham (8 slices per 8-oz pkg)									
784	Regular	2 slices	57	65	104	10	6	1.9	2.8	0.7
785	Extra lean	2 slices	57	71	75	11	3	0.9	1.3	0.3
	Frankfurter (10 per 1-lb pkg), heated									
786	Beef and pork	1 frank	45	54	144	5	13	4.8	6.2	1.2
787	Beef	1 frank	45	55	142	5	13	5.4	6.1	0.6
	Pork sausage, fresh, cooked									
788	Link (4" x ⅞" raw)	2 links	26	45	96	5	8	2.8	3.6	1.0
789	Patty (3⅞" x ¼" raw)	1 patty	27	45	100	5	8	2.9	3.8	1.0
	Salami, beef and pork									
790	Cooked type (8 slices per 8-oz pkg)	2 slices	57	60	143	8	11	4.6	5.2	1.2
791	Dry type, slice, 3⅛" x 1⁄16"	2 slices	20	35	84	5	7	2.4	3.4	0.6
792	Sandwich spread (pork, beef)	1 tbsp	15	60	35	1	3	0.9	1.1	0.4
793	Vienna sausage (7 per 4-oz can)	1 sausage	16	60	45	2	4	1.5	2.0	0.3
	Veal, lean and fat, cooked									
794	Cutlet, braised, 4⅛" x 2¼" x ½"	3 oz	85	55	179	31	5	2.2	2.0	0.4
795	Rib, roasted, 2 pieces, 4⅛" x 2¼" x ¼"	3 oz	85	60	194	20	12	4.6	4.6	0.8
	Mixed Dishes and Fast Foods									
	Mixed dishes									
796	Beef macaroni, frozen, HEALTHY CHOICE	1 package	240	78	211	14	2	0.7	1.2	0.3
797	Beef stew, canned	1 cup	232	82	218	11	12	5.2	5.5	0.5
798	Chicken pot pie, frozen	1 small pie	217	60	484	13	29	9.7	12.5	4.5
799	Chili con carne with beans, canned	1 cup	222	74	255	20	8	2.1	2.2	1.4
800	Macaroni and cheese, canned, made with corn oil	1 cup	252	82	199	8	6	3.0	NA	1.3
801	Meatless burger crumbles, MORNINGSTAR FARMS	1 cup	110	60	231	22	13	3.3	4.6	4.9
802	Meatless burger patty, frozen, MORNINGSTAR FARMS	1 patty	85	71	91	14	1	0.1	0.3	0.2
803	Pasta with meatballs in tomato sauce, canned	1 cup	252	78	260	11	10	4.0	4.2	0.6
804	Spaghetti bolognese (meat sauce), frozen, HEALTHY CHOICE	1 package	283	78	255	14	3	1.0	0.9	0.9
805	Spaghetti in tomato sauce with cheese, canned	1 cup	252	80	192	6	2	0.7	0.3	0.3
806	Spinach souffle, home-prepared	1 cup	136	74	219	11	18	7.1	6.8	3.1
807	Tortellini, pasta with cheese filling, frozen	¾ cup (yields 1 cup cooked)	81	31	249	11	6	2.9	1.7	0.4

Mixed Dishes and Fast Foods (continued)

Food No.	Food Description	Measure of edible portion	Weight (g)	Water (%)	Calories (kcal)	Protein (g)	Total fat (g)	Fatty acids: Saturated (g)	Fatty acids: Monounsaturated (g)	Fatty acids: Polyunsaturated (g)
	Fast foods									
	Breakfast items									
808	Biscuit with egg and sausage	1 biscuit	180	43	581	19	39	15.0	16.4	4.4
809	Croissant with egg, cheese, bacon	1 croissant	129	44	413	16	28	15.4	9.2	1.8
	Danish pastry									
810	Cheese filled	1 pastry	91	34	353	6	25	5.1	15.6	2.4
811	Fruit filled	1 pastry	94	29	335	5	16	3.3	10.1	1.6
812	English muffin with egg, cheese, Canadian bacon	1 muffin	137	57	289	17	13	4.7	4.7	1.6
813	French toast with butter	2 slices	135	51	356	10	19	7.7	7.1	2.4
814	French toast sticks	5 sticks	141	30	513	8	29	4.7	12.6	9.9
815	Hashed brown potatoes	½ cup	72	60	151	2	9	4.3	3.9	0.5
816	Pancakes with butter, syrup	2 pancakes	232	50	520	8	14	5.9	5.3	2.0
	Burrito									
817	With beans and cheese	1 burrito	93	54	189	8	6	3.4	1.2	0.9
818	With beans and meat	1 burrito	116	52	255	11	9	4.2	3.5	0.6
	Cheeseburger									
	Regular size, with condiments									
819	Double patty with mayo type dressing, vegetables	1 sandwich	166	51	417	21	21	8.7	7.8	2.7
820	Single patty	1 sandwich	113	48	295	16	14	6.3	5.3	1.1
	Regular size, plain									
821	Double patty	1 sandwich	155	42	457	28	28	13.0	11.0	1.9
822	Double patty with 3-piece bun	1 sandwich	160	43	461	22	22	9.5	8.3	1.8
823	Single patty	1 sandwich	102	37	319	15	15	6.5	5.8	1.5
	Large, with condiments									
824	Single patty with mayo type dressing, vegetables	1 sandwich	219	53	563	28	33	15.0	12.6	2.0
825	Single patty with bacon	1 sandwich	195	44	608	32	37	16.2	14.5	2.7
826	Chicken fillet (breaded and fried) sandwich, plain	1 sandwich	182	47	515	24	29	8.5	10.4	8.4
	Chicken, fried. See Poultry and Poultry Products.									
827	Chicken pieces, boneless, breaded and fried, plain	6 pieces	106	47	319	18	21	4.7	10.5	4.6
828	Chili con carne	1 cup	253	77	256	25	8	3.4	3.4	0.5
829	Chimichanga with beef	1 chimichanga	174	51	425	20	20	8.5	8.1	1.1
830	Coleslaw	¾ cup	99	74	147	1	11	1.6	2.4	6.4
	Desserts									
831	Ice milk, soft, vanilla, in cone	1 cone	103	65	164	4	6	3.5	1.8	0.4
832	Pie, fried, with fruit filling (5" x 3¾")	1 pie	128	38	404	4	21	3.1	9.5	6.9
833	Sundae, hot fudge	1 sundae	158	60	284	6	9	5.0	2.3	0.8
834	Enchilada with cheese	1 enchilada	163	63	319	10	19	10.6	6.3	0.8
835	Fish sandwich, with tartar sauce and cheese	1 sandwich	183	45	523	21	29	8.1	8.9	9.4
836	French fries	1 small	85	35	291	4	16	3.3	9.0	2.7
837		1 medium	134	35	458	6	25	5.2	14.3	4.2
838		1 large	169	35	578	7	31	6.5	18.0	5.3
839	Frijoles (refried beans, chili sauce, cheese)	1 cup	167	69	225	11	8	4.1	2.6	0.7

Food No.	Food Description	Measure of edible portion	Weight (g)	Water (%)	Calories (kcal)	Protein (g)	Total fat (g)	Fatty acids: Saturated (g)	Fatty acids: Monounsaturated (g)	Fatty acids: Polyunsaturated (g)

Mixed Dishes and Fast Foods (continued)

Food No.	Food Description	Measure of edible portion	Weight (g)	Water (%)	Calories (kcal)	Protein (g)	Total fat (g)	Saturated (g)	Monounsaturated (g)	Polyunsaturated (g)
	Fast foods (continued)									
	Hamburger									
	Regular size, with condiments									
840	Double patty	1 sandwich	215	51	576	32	32	12.0	14.1	2.8
841	Single patty	1 sandwich	106	45	272	12	10	3.6	3.4	1.0
	Large, with condiments, mayo type dressing, and vegetables									
842	Double patty	1 sandwich	226	54	540	34	27	10.5	10.3	2.8
843	Single patty	1 sandwich	218	56	512	26	27	10.4	11.4	2.2
	Hot dog									
844	Plain	1 sandwich	98	54	242	10	15	5.1	6.9	1.7
845	With chili	1 sandwich	114	48	296	14	13	4.9	6.6	1.2
846	With corn flour coating (corndog)	1 corndog	175	47	460	17	19	5.2	9.1	3.5
847	Hush puppies	5 pieces	78	32	257	5	12	2.7	7.8	0.4
848	Mashed potatoes	⅓ cup	80	79	66	2	1	0.4	0.3	0.2
849	Nachos, with cheese sauce	6-8 nachos	113	40	346	9	19	7.8	8.0	2.2
850	Onion rings, breaded and fried	8-9 rings	83	37	276	4	16	7.0	6.7	0.7
	Pizza (slice = ⅛ of 12" pizza)									
851	Cheese	1 slice	63	48	140	8	3	1.5	1.0	0.5
852	Meat and vegetables	1 slice	79	48	184	13	5	1.5	2.5	0.9
853	Pepperoni	1 slice	71	47	181	10	7	2.2	3.1	1.2
854	Roast beef sandwich, plain	1 sandwich	139	49	346	22	14	3.6	6.8	1.7
855	Salad, tossed, with chicken, no dressing	1½ cups	218	87	105	17	2	0.6	0.7	0.6
856	Salad, tossed, with egg, cheese, no dressing	1½ cups	217	90	102	9	6	3.0	1.8	0.5
	Shake									
857	Chocolate	16 fl oz	333	72	423	11	12	7.7	3.6	0.5
858	Vanilla	16 fl oz	333	75	370	12	10	6.2	2.9	0.4
859	Shrimp, breaded and fried	6-8 shrimp	164	48	454	19	25	5.4	17.4	0.6
	Submarine sandwich (6" long), with oil and vinegar									
860	Cold cuts (with lettuce, cheese, salami, ham, tomato, onion)	1 sandwich	228	58	456	22	19	6.8	8.2	2.3
861	Roast beef (with tomato, lettuce, mayo)	1 sandwich	216	59	410	29	13	7.1	1.8	2.6
862	Tuna salad (with mayo, lettuce)	1 sandwich	256	54	584	30	28	5.3	13.4	7.3
863	Taco, beef	1 small	171	58	369	21	21	11.4	6.6	1.0
864		1 large	263	58	568	32	32	17.5	10.1	1.5
865	Taco salad (with ground beef, cheese, taco shell)	1½ cups	198	72	279	13	15	6.8	5.2	1.7
	Tostada (with cheese, tomato, lettuce)									
866	With beans and beef	1 tostada	225	70	333	16	17	11.5	3.5	0.6
867	With guacamole	1 tostada	131	73	181	6	12	5.0	4.3	1.5

Food No.	Food Description	Measure of edible portion	Weight (g)	Water (%)	Calories (kcal)	Protein (g)	Total fat (g)	Fatty acids: Saturated (g)	Fatty acids: Monounsaturated (g)	Fatty acids: Polyunsaturated (g)

Poultry and Poultry Products

Food No.	Food Description	Measure of edible portion	Weight (g)	Water (%)	Calories (kcal)	Protein (g)	Total fat (g)	Saturated (g)	Monounsaturated (g)	Polyunsaturated (g)
	Chicken									
	Fried in vegetable shortening, meat with skin									
	Batter dipped									
868	Breast, ½ breast (5.6 oz with bones)	½ breast	140	52	364	35	18	4.9	7.6	4.3
869	Drumstick (3.4 oz with bones)	1 drumstick	72	53	193	16	11	3.0	4.6	2.7
870	Thigh	1 thigh	86	52	238	19	14	3.8	5.8	3.4
871	Wing	1 wing	49	46	159	10	11	2.9	4.4	2.5
	Flour coated									
872	Breast, ½ breast (4.2 oz with bones)	½ breast	98	57	218	31	9	2.4	3.4	1.9
873	Drumstick (2.6 oz with bones)	1 drumstick	49	57	120	13	7	1.8	2.7	1.6
	Fried, meat only									
874	Dark meat	3 oz	85	56	203	25	10	2.7	3.7	2.4
875	Light meat	3 oz	85	60	163	28	5	1.3	1.7	1.1
	Roasted, meat only									
876	Breast, ½ breast (4.2 oz with bone and skin)	½ breast	86	65	142	27	3	0.9	1.1	0.7
877	Drumstick (2.9 oz with bone and skin)	1 drumstick	44	67	76	12	2	0.7	0.8	0.6
878	Thigh	1 thigh	52	63	109	13	6	1.6	2.2	1.3
879	Stewed, meat only, light and dark meat, chopped or diced	1 cup	140	56	332	43	17	4.3	5.7	4.0
880	Chicken giblets, simmered, chopped	1 cup	145	68	228	37	7	2.2	1.7	1.6
881	Chicken liver, simmered	1 liver	20	68	31	5	1	0.4	0.3	0.2
882	Chicken neck, meat only, simmered	1 neck	18	67	32	4	1	0.4	0.5	0.4
883	Duck, roasted, flesh only	½ duck	221	64	444	52	25	9.2	8.2	3.2
	Turkey									
	Roasted, meat only									
884	Dark meat	3 oz	85	63	159	24	6	2.1	1.4	1.8
885	Light meat	3 oz	85	66	133	25	3	0.9	0.5	0.7
886	Light and dark meat, chopped or diced	1 cup	140	65	238	41	7	2.3	1.4	2.0
	Ground, cooked									
887	Patty, from 4 oz raw	1 patty	82	59	193	22	11	2.8	4.0	2.6
888	Crumbled	1 cup	127	59	298	35	17	4.3	6.2	4.1
889	Turkey giblets, simmered, chopped	1 cup	145	65	242	39	7	2.2	1.7	1.7
890	Turkey neck, meat only, simmered	1 neck	152	65	274	41	11	3.7	2.5	3.3
	Poultry food products									
	Chicken									
891	Canned, boneless	5 oz	142	69	234	31	11	3.1	4.5	2.5
892	Frankfurter (10 per 1 lb pkg)	1 frank	45	58	116	6	9	2.5	3.8	1.8
893	Roll, light meat (6 slices per 6-oz pkg)	2 slices	57	69	90	11	4	1.1	1.7	0.9

Food No.	Food Description	Measure of edible portion	Weight (g)	Water (%)	Calories (kcal)	Protein (g)	Total fat (g)	Fatty acids: Saturated (g)	Fatty acids: Monounsaturated (g)	Fatty acids: Polyunsaturated (g)

Poultry and Poultry Products (continued)

Food No.	Food Description	Measure of edible portion	Weight (g)	Water (%)	Calories (kcal)	Protein (g)	Total fat (g)	Saturated (g)	Monounsaturated (g)	Polyunsaturated (g)
	Poultry food products (continued)									
	Turkey									
894	Gravy and turkey, frozen	5-oz package	142	85	95	8	4	1.2	1.4	0.7
895	Patties, breaded or battered, fried (2.25 oz)	1 patty	64	50	181	9	12	3.0	4.8	3.0
896	Roast, boneless, frozen, seasoned, light and dark meat, cooked	3 oz	85	68	132	18	5	1.6	1.0	1.4

Soups, Sauces, and Gravies

Food No.	Food Description	Measure of edible portion	Weight (g)	Water (%)	Calories (kcal)	Protein (g)	Total fat (g)	Saturated (g)	Monounsaturated (g)	Polyunsaturated (g)
	Soups									
	Canned, condensed									
	Prepared with equal volume of whole milk									
897	Clam chowder, New England	1 cup	248	85	164	9	7	3.0	2.3	1.1
898	Cream of chicken	1 cup	248	85	191	7	11	4.6	4.5	1.6
899	Cream of mushroom	1 cup	248	85	203	6	14	5.1	3.0	4.6
900	Tomato	1 cup	248	85	161	6	6	2.9	1.6	1.1
	Prepared with equal volume of water									
901	Bean with pork	1 cup	253	84	172	8	6	1.5	2.2	1.8
902	Beef broth, bouillon, consomme	1 cup	241	96	29	5	0	0.0	0.0	0.0
903	Beef noodle	1 cup	244	92	83	5	3	1.1	1.2	0.5
904	Chicken noodle	1 cup	241	92	75	4	2	0.7	1.1	0.6
905	Chicken and rice	1 cup	241	94	60	4	2	0.5	0.9	0.4
906	Clam chowder, Manhattan	1 cup	244	92	78	2	2	0.4	0.4	1.3
907	Cream of chicken	1 cup	244	91	117	3	7	2.1	3.3	1.5
908	Cream of mushroom	1 cup	244	90	129	2	9	2.4	1.7	4.2
909	Minestrone	1 cup	241	91	82	4	3	0.6	0.7	1.1
910	Pea, green	1 cup	250	83	165	9	3	1.4	1.0	0.4
911	Tomato	1 cup	244	90	85	2	2	0.4	0.4	1.0
912	Vegetable beef	1 cup	244	92	78	6	2	0.9	0.8	0.1
913	Vegetarian vegetable	1 cup	241	92	72	2	2	0.3	0.8	0.7
	Canned, ready to serve, chunky									
914	Bean with ham	1 cup	243	79	231	13	9	3.3	3.8	0.9
915	Chicken noodle	1 cup	240	84	175	13	6	1.4	2.7	1.5
916	Chicken and vegetable	1 cup	240	83	166	12	5	1.4	2.2	1.0
917	Vegetable	1 cup	240	88	122	4	4	0.6	1.6	1.4
	Canned, ready to serve, low fat, reduced sodium									
918	Chicken broth	1 cup	240	97	17	3	0	0.0	0.0	0.0
919	Chicken noodle	1 cup	237	92	76	6	2	0.4	0.6	0.4
920	Chicken and rice	1 cup	241	88	116	7	3	0.9	1.3	0.7
921	Chicken and rice with vegetables	1 cup	239	91	88	6	1	0.4	0.5	0.5
922	Clam chowder, New England	1 cup	244	89	117	5	2	0.5	0.7	0.4
923	Lentil	1 cup	242	88	126	8	2	0.3	0.8	0.2
924	Minestrone	1 cup	241	87	123	5	3	0.4	0.9	1.0
925	Vegetable	1 cup	238	91	81	4	1	0.3	0.4	0.3

Table 9. Nutritive Value of the Edible Part of Food

Soups, Sauces, and Gravies (continued)

Food No.	Food Description	Measure of edible portion	Weight (g)	Water (%)	Calories (kcal)	Protein (g)	Total fat (g)	Fatty acids: Saturated (g)	Fatty acids: Monounsaturated (g)	Fatty acids: Polyunsaturated (g)
	Soups (continued)									
	Dehydrated									
	Unprepared									
926	Beef bouillon	1 packet	6	3	14	1	1	0.3	0.2	Tr
927	Onion	1 packet	39	4	115	5	2	0.5	1.4	0.3
	Prepared with water									
928	Chicken noodle	1 cup	252	94	58	2	1	0.3	0.5	0.4
929	Onion	1 cup	246	96	27	1	1	0.1	0.3	0.1
	Home prepared, stock									
930	Beef	1 cup	240	96	31	5	Tr	0.1	0.1	Tr
931	Chicken	1 cup	240	92	86	6	3	0.8	1.4	0.5
932	Fish	1 cup	233	97	40	5	2	0.5	0.5	0.3
	Sauces									
	Home recipe									
933	Cheese	1 cup	243	67	479	25	36	19.5	11.5	3.4
934	White, medium, made with whole milk	1 cup	250	75	368	10	27	7.1	11.1	7.2
	Ready to serve									
935	Barbecue	1 tbsp	16	81	12	Tr	Tr	Tr	0.1	0.1
936	Cheese	¼ cup	63	71	110	4	8	3.8	2.4	1.6
937	Hoisin	1 tbsp	16	44	35	1	1	0.1	0.2	0.3
938	Nacho cheese	¼ cup	63	70	119	5	10	4.2	3.1	2.1
939	Pepper or hot	1 tsp	5	90	1	Tr	Tr	Tr	Tr	Tr
940	Salsa	1 tbsp	16	90	4	Tr	Tr	Tr	Tr	Tr
941	Soy	1 tbsp	16	69	9	1	Tr	Tr	Tr	Tr
942	Spaghetti/marinara/pasta	1 cup	250	87	143	4	5	0.7	2.2	1.8
943	Teriyaki	1 tbsp	18	68	15	1	0	0.0	0.0	0.0
944	Tomato chili	¼ cup	68	68	71	2	Tr	Tr	Tr	0.1
945	Worcestershire	1 tbsp	17	70	11	0	0	0.0	0.0	0.0
	Gravies, canned									
946	Beef	¼ cup	58	87	31	2	1	0.7	0.6	Tr
947	Chicken	¼ cup	60	85	47	1	3	0.8	1.5	0.9
948	Country sausage	¼ cup	62	75	96	3	8	2.0	2.9	2.2
949	Mushroom	¼ cup	60	89	30	1	2	0.2	0.7	0.6
950	Turkey	¼ cup	60	89	31	2	1	0.4	0.5	0.3

Sugars and Sweets

Food No.	Food Description	Measure of edible portion	Weight (g)	Water (%)	Calories (kcal)	Protein (g)	Total fat (g)	Fatty acids: Saturated (g)	Fatty acids: Monounsaturated (g)	Fatty acids: Polyunsaturated (g)
	Candy									
951	BUTTERFINGER (NESTLE)	1 fun size bar	7	2	34	1	1	0.7	0.4	0.2
	Caramel									
952	Plain	1 piece	10	9	39	Tr	1	0.7	0.1	Tr
953	Chocolate flavored roll	1 piece	7	7	25	Tr	Tr	Tr	0.1	0.1
954	Carob	1 oz	28	2	153	2	9	8.2	0.1	0.1
	Chocolate, milk									
955	Plain	1 bar (1.55 oz)	44	1	226	3	14	8.1	4.4	0.5
956	With almonds	1 bar (1.45 oz)	41	2	216	4	14	7.0	5.5	0.9
957	With peanuts, MR. GOODBAR (HERSHEY)	1 bar (1.75 oz)	49	1	267	5	17	7.3	5.7	2.4
958	With rice cereal, NESTLE CRUNCH	1 bar (1.55 oz)	44	1	230	3	12	6.7	3.8	0.4
	Chocolate chips									
959	Milk	1 cup	168	1	862	12	52	31.0	16.7	1.8
960	Semisweet	1 cup	168	1	805	7	50	29.8	16.7	1.6
961	White	1 cup	170	1	916	10	55	33.0	15.5	1.7
962	Chocolate coated peanuts	10 pieces	40	2	208	5	13	5.8	5.2	1.7
963	Chocolate coated raisins	10 pieces	10	11	39	Tr	1	0.9	0.5	0.1
964	Fruit leather, pieces	1 oz	28	12	97	Tr	2	0.3	0.9	0.8

Food No.	Food Description	Measure of edible portion	Weight (g)	Water (%)	Calories (kcal)	Protein (g)	Total fat (g)	Fatty acids Saturated (g)	Fatty acids Monounsaturated (g)	Fatty acids Polyunsaturated (g)

Sugars and Sweets (continued)

Food No.	Food Description	Measure of edible portion	Weight (g)	Water (%)	Calories (kcal)	Protein (g)	Total fat (g)	Saturated (g)	Monounsaturated (g)	Polyunsaturated (g)
	Candy (continued)									
965	Fruit leather, rolls	1 large	21	11	74	Tr	1	0.1	0.3	0.1
966		1 small	14	11	49	Tr	Tr	0.1	0.2	0.1
	Fudge, prepared from recipe									
	Chocolate									
967	Plain	1 piece	17	10	65	Tr	1	0.9	0.4	0.1
968	With nuts	1 piece	19	7	81	1	3	1.1	0.8	1.0
	Vanilla									
969	Plain	1 piece	16	11	59	Tr	1	0.5	0.2	Tr
970	With nuts	1 piece	15	8	62	Tr	2	0.6	0.5	0.8
	Gumdrops/gummy candies									
971	Gumdrops (¾" dia)	1 cup	182	1	703	0	0	0.0	0.0	0.0
972		1 medium	4	1	16	0	0	0.0	0.0	0.0
973	Gummy bears	10 bears	22	1	85	0	0	0.0	0.0	0.0
974	Gummy worms	10 worms	74	1	286	0	0	0.0	0.0	0.0
975	Hard candy	1 piece	6	1	24	0	Tr	0.0	0.0	0.0
976		1 small piece	3	1	12	0	Tr	0.0	0.0	0.0
977	Jelly beans	10 large	28	6	104	0	Tr	Tr	0.1	Tr
978		10 small	11	6	40	0	Tr	Tr	Tr	Tr
979	KIT KAT (HERSHEY)	1 bar (1.5 oz)	42	2	216	3	11	6.8	3.1	0.3
	Marshmallows									
980	Miniature	1 cup	50	16	159	1	Tr	Tr	Tr	Tr
981	Regular	1 regular	7	16	23	Tr	Tr	Tr	Tr	Tr
	M&M's (M&M MARS)									
982	Peanut	¼ cup	43	2	222	4	11	4.4	4.7	1.8
983		10 pieces	20	2	103	2	5	2.1	2.2	0.8
984	Plain	¼ cup	52	2	256	2	11	6.8	3.6	0.3
985		10 pieces	7	2	34	Tr	1	0.9	0.5	Tr
986	MILKY WAY (M&M MARS)	1 fun size bar	18	6	76	1	3	1.4	1.1	0.1
987		1 bar (2.15 oz)	61	6	258	3	10	4.8	3.7	0.4
988	REESE'S Peanut butter cup (HERSHEY)	1 miniature cup	7	2	38	1	2	0.8	0.9	0.4
989		1 package (contains 2)	45	2	243	5	14	5.0	5.9	2.5
990	SNICKERS bar (M&M MARS)	1 fun size bar	15	5	72	1	4	1.3	1.6	0.7
991		1 king size bar (4 oz)	113	5	541	9	28	10.2	11.8	5.6
992		1 bar (2 oz)	57	5	273	5	14	5.1	6.0	2.8
993	SPECIAL DARK sweet chocolate (HERSHEY)	1 miniature	8	1	46	Tr	3	1.7	0.9	0.1
994	STARBURST fruit chews (M&M MARS)	1 piece	5	7	20	Tr	Tr	0.1	0.2	0.2
995		1 package (2.07 oz)	59	7	234	Tr	5	0.7	2.1	1.8
	Frosting, ready to eat									
996	Chocolate	1/12 package	38	17	151	Tr	7	2.1	3.4	0.8
997	Vanilla	1/12 package	38	13	159	Tr	6	1.9	3.3	0.9
	Frozen desserts (nondairy)									
998	Fruit and juice bar	1 bar (2.5 fl oz)	77	78	63	1	Tr	0.0	0.0	Tr
999	Ice pop	1 bar (2 fl oz)	59	80	42	0	0	0.0	0.0	0.0
1000	Italian ices	½ cup	116	86	61	Tr	Tr	0.0	0.0	0.0
1001	Fruit butter, apple	1 tbsp	17	56	29	Tr	0	0.0	0.0	0.0
	Gelatin dessert, prepared with gelatin dessert powder and water									
1002	Regular	½ cup	135	85	80	2	0	0.0	0.0	0.0
1003	Reduced calorie (with aspartame)	½ cup	117	98	8	1	0	0.0	0.0	0.0

Food No.	Food Description	Measure of edible portion	Weight (g)	Water (%)	Calories (kcal)	Protein (g)	Total fat (g)	Fatty acids: Saturated (g)	Fatty acids: Monounsaturated (g)	Fatty acids: Polyunsaturated (g)

Sugars and Sweets (continued)

Food No.	Food Description	Measure of edible portion	Weight (g)	Water (%)	Calories (kcal)	Protein (g)	Total fat (g)	Saturated (g)	Monounsaturated (g)	Polyunsaturated (g)
1004	Honey, strained or extracted	1 tbsp	21	17	64	Tr	0	0.0	0.0	0.0
1005		1 cup	339	17	1,031	1	0	0.0	0.0	0.0
1006	Jams and preserves	1 tbsp	20	30	56	Tr	Tr	Tr	Tr	0.0
1007		1 packet (0.5 oz)	14	30	39	Tr	Tr	Tr	Tr	0.0
1008	Jellies	1 tbsp	19	29	54	Tr	Tr	Tr	Tr	Tr
1009		1 packet (0.5 oz)	14	29	40	Tr	Tr	Tr	Tr	Tr
	Puddings									
	Prepared with dry mix and 2% milk									
	Chocolate									
1010	Instant	½ cup	147	75	150	5	3	1.6	0.9	0.2
1011	Regular (cooked)	½ cup	142	74	151	5	3	1.8	0.8	0.1
	Vanilla									
1012	Instant	½ cup	142	75	148	4	2	1.4	0.7	0.1
1013	Regular (cooked)	½ cup	140	76	141	4	2	1.5	0.7	0.1
	Ready to eat									
	Regular									
1014	Chocolate	4 oz	113	69	150	3	5	0.8	1.9	1.6
1015	Rice	4 oz	113	68	184	2	8	1.3	3.6	3.2
1016	Tapioca	4 oz	113	74	134	2	4	0.7	1.8	1.5
1017	Vanilla	4 oz	113	71	147	3	4	0.6	1.7	1.5
	Fat free									
1018	Chocolate	4 oz	113	76	107	3	Tr	0.3	0.1	Tr
1019	Tapioca	4 oz	113	77	98	2	Tr	0.1	Tr	Tr
1020	Vanilla	4 oz	113	76	105	2	Tr	0.1	Tr	Tr
	Sugar									
	Brown									
1021	Packed	1 cup	220	2	827	0	0	0.0	0.0	0.0
1022	Unpacked	1 cup	145	2	545	0	0	0.0	0.0	0.0
1023		1 tbsp	9	2	34	0	0	0.0	0.0	0.0
	White									
1024	Granulated	1 packet	6	0	23	0	0	0.0	0.0	0.0
1025		1 tsp	4	0	16	0	0	0.0	0.0	0.0
1026		1 cup	200	0	774	0	0	0.0	0.0	0.0
1027	Powdered, unsifted	1 tbsp	8	Tr	31	0	Tr	Tr	Tr	Tr
1028		1 cup	120	Tr	467	0	Tr	Tr	Tr	0.1
	Syrup									
	Chocolate flavored syrup or topping									
1029	Thin type	1 tbsp	19	31	53	Tr	Tr	0.1	0.1	Tr
1030	Fudge type	1 tbsp	19	22	67	1	2	0.8	0.7	0.1
1031	Corn, light	1 tbsp	20	23	56	0	0	0.0	0.0	0.0
1032	Maple	1 tbsp	20	32	52	0	Tr	Tr	Tr	Tr
1033	Molasses, blackstrap	1 tbsp	20	29	47	0	0	0.0	0.0	0.0
1034		1 cup	328	29	771	0	0	0.0	0.0	0.0
	Table blend, pancake									
1035	Regular	1 tbsp	20	24	57	0	0	0.0	0.0	0.0
1036	Reduced calorie	1 tbsp	15	55	25	0	0	0.0	0.0	0.0

Food No.	Food Description	Measure of edible portion	Weight (g)	Water (%)	Calories (kcal)	Protein (g)	Total fat (g)	Fatty acids Saturated (g)	Monounsaturated (g)	Polyunsaturated (g)

Vegetables and Vegetable Products

Food No.	Food Description	Measure of edible portion	Weight (g)	Water (%)	Calories (kcal)	Protein (g)	Total fat (g)	Saturated (g)	Monounsaturated (g)	Polyunsaturated (g)
1037	Alfalfa sprouts, raw	1 cup	33	91	10	1	Tr	Tr	Tr	0.1
1038	Artichokes, globe or French, cooked, drained	1 cup	168	84	84	6	Tr	0.1	Tr	0.1
1039		1 medium	120	84	60	4	Tr	Tr	Tr	0.1
	Asparagus, green									
	Cooked, drained									
1040	From raw	1 cup	180	92	43	5	1	0.1	Tr	0.2
1041		4 spears	60	92	14	2	Tr	Tr	Tr	0.1
1042	From frozen	1 cup	180	91	50	5	1	0.2	Tr	0.3
1043		4 spears	60	91	17	2	Tr	0.1	Tr	0.1
1044	Canned, spears, about 5" long, drained	1 cup	242	94	46	5	2	0.4	0.1	0.7
1045		4 spears	72	94	14	2	Tr	0.1	Tr	0.2
1046	Bamboo shoots, canned, drained	1 cup	131	94	25	2	1	0.1	Tr	0.2
	Beans									
	Lima, immature seeds, frozen, cooked, drained									
1047	Ford hooks	1 cup	170	74	170	10	1	0.1	Tr	0.3
1048	Baby limas	1 cup	180	72	189	12	1	0.1	Tr	0.3
	Snap, cut									
	Cooked, drained									
	From raw									
1049	Green	1 cup	125	89	44	2	Tr	0.1	Tr	0.2
1050	Yellow	1 cup	125	89	44	2	Tr	0.1	Tr	0.2
	From frozen									
1051	Green	1 cup	135	91	38	2	Tr	0.1	Tr	0.1
1052	Yellow	1 cup	135	91	38	2	Tr	0.1	Tr	0.1
	Canned, drained									
1053	Green	1 cup	135	93	27	2	Tr	Tr	Tr	0.1
1054	Yellow	1 cup	135	93	27	2	Tr	Tr	Tr	0.1
	Beans, dry. See Legumes.									
	Bean sprouts (mung)									
1055	Raw	1 cup	104	90	31	3	Tr	Tr	Tr	0.1
1056	Cooked, drained	1 cup	124	93	26	3	Tr	Tr	Tr	Tr
	Beets									
	Cooked, drained									
1057	Slices	1 cup	170	87	75	3	Tr	Tr	0.1	0.1
1058	Whole beet, 2" dia	1 beet	50	87	22	1	Tr	Tr	Tr	Tr
	Canned, drained									
1059	Slices	1 cup	170	91	53	2	Tr	Tr	Tr	0.1
1060	Whole beet	1 beet	24	91	7	Tr	Tr	Tr	Tr	Tr
1061	Beet greens, leaves and stems, cooked, drained, 1" pieces	1 cup	144	89	39	4	Tr	Tr	0.1	0.1
	Black eyed peas, immature seeds, cooked, drained									
1062	From raw	1 cup	165	75	160	5	1	0.2	0.1	0.3
1063	From frozen	1 cup	170	66	224	14	1	0.3	0.1	0.5
	Broccoli									
	Raw									
1064	Chopped or diced	1 cup	88	91	25	3	Tr	Tr	Tr	0.1
1065	Spear, about 5" long	1 spear	31	91	9	1	Tr	Tr	Tr	0.1
1066	Flower cluster	1 floweret	11	91	3	Tr	Tr	Tr	Tr	Tr
	Cooked, drained									
	From raw									
1067	Chopped	1 cup	156	91	44	5	1	0.1	Tr	0.3
1068	Spear, about 5" long	1 spear	37	91	10	1	Tr	Tr	Tr	0.1
1069	From frozen, chopped	1 cup	184	91	52	6	Tr	Tr	Tr	0.1

Table 9. Nutritive Value of the Edible Part of Food

Food No.	Food Description	Measure of edible portion	Weight (g)	Water (%)	Calories (kcal)	Protein (g)	Total fat (g)	Fatty acids Saturated (g)	Fatty acids Monounsaturated (g)	Fatty acids Polyunsaturated (g)

Vegetables and Vegetable Products (continued)

Food No.	Food Description	Measure of edible portion	Weight (g)	Water (%)	Calories (kcal)	Protein (g)	Total fat (g)	Saturated (g)	Monounsaturated (g)	Polyunsaturated (g)
	Brussels sprouts, cooked, drained									
1070	From raw	1 cup	156	87	61	4	1	0.2	0.1	0.4
1071	From frozen	1 cup	155	87	65	6	1	0.1	Tr	0.3
	Cabbage, common varieties, shredded									
1072	Raw	1 cup	70	92	18	1	Tr	Tr	Tr	0.1
1073	Cooked, drained	1 cup	150	94	33	2	1	0.1	Tr	0.3
	Cabbage, Chinese, shredded, cooked, drained									
1074	Pak choi or bok choy	1 cup	170	96	20	3	Tr	Tr	Tr	0.1
1075	Pe tsai	1 cup	119	95	17	2	Tr	Tr	Tr	0.1
1076	Cabbage, red, raw, shredded	1 cup	70	92	19	1	Tr	Tr	Tr	0.1
1077	Cabbage, savoy, raw, shredded	1 cup	70	91	19	1	Tr	Tr	Tr	Tr
1078	Carrot juice, canned	1 cup	236	89	94	2	Tr	0.1	Tr	0.2
	Carrots									
	Raw									
1079	Whole, 7½" long	1 carrot	72	88	31	1	Tr	Tr	Tr	0.1
1080	Grated	1 cup	110	88	47	1	Tr	Tr	Tr	0.1
1081	Baby	1 medium	10	90	4	Tr	Tr	Tr	Tr	Tr
	Cooked, sliced, drained									
1082	From raw	1 cup	156	87	70	2	Tr	0.1	Tr	0.1
1083	From frozen	1 cup	146	90	53	2	Tr	Tr	Tr	0.1
1084	Canned, sliced, drained	1 cup	146	93	37	1	Tr	0.1	Tr	0.1
	Cauliflower									
1085	Raw	1 floweret	13	92	3	Tr	Tr	Tr	Tr	Tr
1086		1 cup	100	92	25	2	Tr	Tr	Tr	0.1
	Cooked, drained, 1" pieces									
1087	From raw	1 cup	124	93	29	2	1	0.1	Tr	0.3
1088		3 flowerets	54	93	12	1	Tr	Tr	Tr	0.1
1089	From frozen	1 cup	180	94	34	3	Tr	0.1	Tr	0.2
	Celery									
	Raw									
1090	Stalk, 7½ to 8" long	1 stalk	40	95	6	Tr	Tr	Tr	Tr	Tr
1091	Pieces, diced	1 cup	120	95	19	1	Tr	Tr	Tr	0.1
	Cooked, drained									
1092	Stalk, medium	1 stalk	38	94	7	Tr	Tr	Tr	Tr	Tr
1093	Pieces, diced	1 cup	150	94	27	1	Tr	0.1	Tr	0.1
1094	Chives, raw, chopped	1 tbsp	3	91	1	Tr	Tr	Tr	Tr	Tr
1095	Cilantro, raw	1 tsp	2	92	Tr	Tr	Tr	Tr	Tr	Tr
1096	Coleslaw, home prepared	1 cup	120	82	83	2	3	0.5	0.8	1.6
	Collards, cooked, drained, chopped									
1097	From raw	1 cup	190	92	49	4	1	0.1	Tr	0.3
1098	From frozen	1 cup	170	88	61	5	1	0.1	Tr	0.4
	Corn, sweet, yellow									
	Cooked, drained									
1099	From raw, kernels on cob	1 ear	77	70	83	3	1	0.2	0.3	0.5
	From frozen									
1100	Kernels on cob	1 ear	63	73	59	2	Tr	0.1	0.1	0.2
1101	Kernels	1 cup	164	77	131	5	1	0.1	0.2	0.3
	Canned									
1102	Cream style	1 cup	256	79	184	4	1	0.2	0.3	0.5
1103	Whole kernel, vacuum pack	1 cup	210	77	166	5	1	0.2	0.3	0.5
1104	Corn, sweet, white, cooked, drained	1 ear	77	70	83	3	1	0.2	0.3	0.5

*White varieties contain only a trace amount of vitamin A; other nutrients are the same.

Food No.	Food Description	Measure of edible portion	Weight (g)	Water (%)	Calories (kcal)	Protein (g)	Total fat (g)	Fatty acids Saturated (g)	Fatty acids Monounsaturated (g)	Fatty acids Polyunsaturated (g)

Vegetables and Vegetable Products (continued)

Food No.	Food Description	Measure of edible portion	Weight (g)	Water (%)	Calories (kcal)	Protein (g)	Total fat (g)	Saturated (g)	Monounsaturated (g)	Polyunsaturated (g)
	Cucumber									
	Peeled									
1105	Sliced	1 cup	119	96	14	1	Tr	Tr	Tr	0.1
1106	Whole, 8¼" long	1 large	280	96	34	2	Tr	0.1	Tr	0.2
	Unpeeled									
1107	Sliced	1 cup	104	96	14	1	Tr	Tr	Tr	0.1
1108	Whole, 8¼" long	1 large	301	96	39	2	Tr	0.1	Tr	0.2
1109	Dandelion greens, cooked, drained	1 cup	105	90	35	2	1	0.2	Tr	0.3
1110	Dill weed, raw	5 sprigs	1	86	Tr	Tr	Tr	Tr	Tr	Tr
1111	Eggplant, cooked, drained	1 cup	99	92	28	1	Tr	Tr	Tr	0.1
1112	Endive, curly (including escarole), raw, small pieces	1 cup	50	94	9	1	Tr	Tr	Tr	Tr
1113	Garlic, raw	1 clove	3	59	4	Tr	Tr	Tr	Tr	Tr
1114	Hearts of palm, canned	1 piece	33	90	9	1	Tr	Tr	Tr	0.1
1115	Jerusalem artichoke, raw, sliced	1 cup	150	78	114	3	Tr	0.0	Tr	Tr
	Kale, cooked, drained, chopped									
1116	From raw	1 cup	130	91	36	2	1	0.1	Tr	0.3
1117	From frozen	1 cup	130	91	39	4	1	0.1	Tr	0.3
1118	Kohlrabi, cooked, drained, slices	1 cup	165	90	48	3	Tr	Tr	Tr	0.1
1119	Leeks, bulb and lower leaf portion, chopped or diced, cooked, drained	1 cup	104	91	32	1	Tr	Tr	Tr	0.1
	Lettuce, raw									
	Butterhead, as Boston types									
1120	Leaf	1 medium leaf	8	96	1	Tr	Tr	Tr	Tr	Tr
1121	Head, 5" dia	1 head	163	96	21	2	Tr	Tr	Tr	0.2
	Crisphead, as iceberg									
1122	Leaf	1 medium	8	96	1	Tr	Tr	Tr	Tr	Tr
1123	Head, 6" dia	1 head	539	96	65	5	1	0.1	Tr	0.5
1124	Pieces, shredded or chopped	1 cup	55	96	7	1	Tr	Tr	Tr	0.1
	Looseleaf									
1125	Leaf	1 leaf	10	94	2	Tr	Tr	Tr	Tr	Tr
1126	Pieces, shredded	1 cup	56	94	10	1	Tr	Tr	Tr	0.1
	Romaine or cos									
1127	Innerleaf	1 leaf	10	95	1	Tr	Tr	Tr	Tr	Tr
1128	Pieces, shredded	1 cup	56	95	8	1	Tr	Tr	Tr	0.1
	Mushrooms									
1129	Raw, pieces or slices	1 cup	70	92	18	2	Tr	Tr	Tr	0.1
1130	Cooked, drained, pieces	1 cup	156	91	42	3	1	0.1	Tr	0.3
1131	Canned, drained, pieces	1 cup	156	91	37	3	Tr	0.1	Tr	0.2
	Mushrooms, shiitake									
1132	Cooked pieces	1 cup	145	83	80	2	Tr	0.1	0.1	Tr
1133	Dried	1 mushroom	4	10	11	Tr	Tr	Tr	Tr	Tr
1134	Mustard greens, cooked, drained	1 cup	140	94	21	3	Tr	Tr	0.2	0.1
	Okra, sliced, cooked, drained									
1135	From raw	1 cup	160	90	51	3	Tr	0.1	Tr	0.1
1136	From frozen	1 cup	184	91	52	4	1	0.1	0.1	0.1
	Onions									
	Raw									
1137	Chopped	1 cup	160	90	61	2	Tr	Tr	Tr	0.1
1138	Whole, medium, 2½" dia	1 whole	110	90	42	1	Tr	Tr	Tr	0.1
1139	Slice, ⅛" thick	1 slice	14	90	5	Tr	Tr	Tr	Tr	Tr

Vegetables and Vegetable Products (continued)

Food No.	Food Description	Measure of edible portion	Weight (g)	Water (%)	Calories (kcal)	Protein (g)	Total fat (g)	Fatty acids: Saturated (g)	Fatty acids: Monounsaturated (g)	Fatty acids: Polyunsaturated (g)
1140	Cooked (whole or sliced), drained	1 cup	210	88	92	3	Tr	0.1	0.1	0.2
1141		1 medium	94	88	41	1	Tr	Tr	Tr	0.1
1142	Dehydrated flakes	1 tbsp	5	4	17	Tr	Tr	Tr	Tr	Tr
	Onions, spring, raw, top and bulb									
1143	Chopped	1 cup	100	90	32	2	Tr	Tr	Tr	0.1
1144	Whole, medium, 4⅛" long	1 whole	15	90	5	Tr	Tr	Tr	Tr	Tr
1145	Onion rings, 2"-3" dia, breaded, par fried, frozen, oven heated	10 rings	60	29	244	3	16	5.2	6.5	3.1
1146	Parsley, raw	10 sprigs	10	88	4	Tr	Tr	Tr	Tr	Tr
1147	Parsnips, sliced, cooked, drained	1 cup	156	78	126	2	Tr	0.1	0.2	0.1
	Peas, edible pod, cooked, drained									
1148	From raw	1 cup	160	89	67	5	Tr	0.1	Tr	0.2
1149	From frozen	1 cup	160	87	83	6	1	0.1	0.1	0.3
	Peas, green									
1150	Canned, drained	1 cup	170	82	117	8	1	0.1	0.1	0.3
1151	Frozen, boiled, drained	1 cup	160	80	125	8	Tr	0.1	Tr	0.2
	Peppers									
	Hot chili, raw									
1152	Green	1 pepper	45	88	18	1	Tr	Tr	Tr	Tr
1153	Red	1 pepper	45	88	18	1	Tr	Tr	Tr	Tr
1154	Jalapeno, canned, sliced, solids and liquids	¼ cup	26	89	7	Tr	Tr	Tr	Tr	0.1
	Sweet (2¾" long, 2½" dia)									
	Raw									
	Green									
1155	Chopped	1 cup	149	92	40	1	Tr	Tr	Tr	0.2
1156	Ring (¼" thick)	1 ring	10	92	3	Tr	Tr	Tr	Tr	Tr
1157	Whole (2¾" x 2½")	1 pepper	119	92	32	1	Tr	Tr	Tr	0.1
	Red									
1158	Chopped	1 cup	149	92	40	1	Tr	Tr	Tr	0.2
1159	Whole (2¾" x 2½")	1 pepper	119	92	32	1	Tr	Tr	Tr	0.1
	Cooked, drained, chopped									
1160	Green	1 cup	136	92	38	1	Tr	Tr	Tr	0.1
1161	Red	1 cup	136	92	38	1	Tr	Tr	Tr	0.1
1162	Pimento, canned	1 tbsp	12	93	3	Tr	Tr	Tr	Tr	Tr
	Potatoes									
	Baked (2⅓" x 4¾")									
1163	With skin	1 potato	202	71	220	5	Tr	0.1	Tr	0.1
1164	Flesh only	1 potato	156	75	145	3	Tr	Tr	Tr	0.1
1165	Skin only	1 skin	58	47	115	2	Tr	Tr	Tr	Tr
	Boiled (2½" dia)									
1166	Peeled after boiling	1 potato	136	77	118	3	Tr	Tr	Tr	0.1
1167	Peeled before boiling	1 potato	135	77	116	2	Tr	Tr	Tr	0.1
1168		1 cup	156	77	134	3	Tr	Tr	Tr	0.1
	Potato products, prepared									
	Au gratin									
1169	From dry mix, with whole milk, butter	1 cup	245	79	228	6	10	6.3	2.9	0.3
1170	From home recipe, with butter	1 cup	245	74	323	12	19	11.6	5.3	0.7
1171	French fried, frozen, oven heated	10 strips	50	57	100	2	4	0.6	2.4	0.4

Vegetables and Vegetable Products (continued)

Food No.	Food Description	Measure of edible portion	Weight (g)	Water (%)	Calories (kcal)	Protein (g)	Total fat (g)	Fatty acids Saturated (g)	Fatty acids Monounsaturated (g)	Fatty acids Polyunsaturated (g)
	Potato products, prepared (continued)									
	Hashed brown									
1172	From frozen (about 3" x 1½" x ½")	1 patty	29	56	63	1	3	1.3	1.5	0.4
1173	From home recipe	1 cup	156	62	326	4	22	8.5	9.7	2.5
	Mashed									
1174	From dehydrated flakes (without milk); whole milk, butter, and salt added	1 cup	210	76	237	4	12	7.2	3.3	0.5
	From home recipe									
1175	With whole milk	1 cup	210	78	162	4	1	0.7	0.3	0.1
1176	With whole milk and margarine	1 cup	210	76	223	4	9	2.2	3.7	2.5
1177	Potato pancakes, home prepared	1 pancake	76	47	207	5	12	2.3	3.5	5.0
1178	Potato puffs, from frozen	10 puffs	79	53	175	3	8	4.0	3.4	0.6
1179	Potato salad, home prepared	1 cup	250	76	358	7	21	3.6	6.2	9.3
	Scalloped									
1180	From dry mix, with whole milk, butter	1 cup	245	79	228	5	11	6.5	3.0	0.5
1181	From home recipe, with butter	1 cup	245	81	211	7	9	5.5	2.5	0.4
	Pumpkin									
1182	Cooked, mashed	1 cup	245	94	49	2	Tr	0.1	Tr	Tr
1183	Canned	1 cup	245	90	83	3	1	0.4	0.1	Tr
1184	Radishes, raw (¾" to 1" dia)	1 radish	5	95	1	Tr	Tr	Tr	Tr	Tr
1185	Rutabagas, cooked, drained, cubes	1 cup	170	89	66	2	Tr	Tr	Tr	0.2
1186	Sauerkraut, canned, solids and liquid	1 cup	236	93	45	2	Tr	0.1	Tr	0.1
	Seaweed									
1187	Kelp, raw	2 tbsp	10	82	4	Tr	Tr	Tr	Tr	Tr
1188	Spirulina, dried	1 tbsp	1	5	3	1	Tr	Tr	Tr	Tr
1189	Shallots, raw, chopped	1 tbsp	10	80	7	Tr	Tr	Tr	Tr	Tr
1190	Soybeans, green, cooked, drained	1 cup	180	69	254	22	12	1.3	2.2	5.4
	Spinach									
	Raw									
1191	Chopped	1 cup	30	92	7	1	Tr	Tr	Tr	Tr
1192	Leaf	1 leaf	10	92	2	Tr	Tr	Tr	Tr	Tr
	Cooked, drained									
1193	From raw	1 cup	180	91	41	5	Tr	0.1	Tr	0.2
1194	From frozen (chopped or leaf)	1 cup	190	90	53	6	Tr	0.1	Tr	0.2
1195	Canned, drained	1 cup	214	92	49	6	1	0.2	Tr	0.4
	Squash									
	Summer (all varieties), sliced									
1196	Raw	1 cup	113	94	23	1	Tr	Tr	Tr	0.1
1197	Cooked, drained	1 cup	180	94	36	2	1	0.1	Tr	0.2
1198	Winter (all varieties), baked, cubes	1 cup	205	89	80	2	1	0.3	0.1	0.5
1199	Winter, butternut, frozen, cooked, mashed	1 cup	240	88	94	3	Tr	Tr	Tr	0.1
	Sweetpotatoes									
	Cooked (2" dia, 5" long raw)									
1200	Baked, with skin	1 potato	146	73	150	3	Tr	Tr	Tr	0.1
1201	Boiled, without skin	1 potato	156	73	164	3	Tr	0.1	Tr	0.2

Food No.	Food Description	Measure of edible portion	Weight (g)	Water (%)	Calories (kcal)	Protein (g)	Total fat (g)	Fatty acids Saturated (g)	Monounsaturated (g)	Polyunsaturated (g)

Vegetables and Vegetable Products (continued)

Food No.	Food Description	Measure of edible portion	Weight (g)	Water (%)	Calories (kcal)	Protein (g)	Total fat (g)	Saturated (g)	Monounsaturated (g)	Polyunsaturated (g)
	Sweetpotatoes (continued)									
1202	Candied (2½" x 2" piece)	1 piece	105	67	144	1	3	1.4	0.7	0.2
	Canned									
1203	Syrup pack, drained	1 cup	196	72	212	3	1	0.1	Tr	0.3
1204	Vacuum pack, mashed	1 cup	255	76	232	4	1	0.1	Tr	0.2
1205	Tomatillos, raw	1 medium	34	92	11	Tr	Tr	Tr	0.1	0.1
	Tomatoes									
	Raw, year round average									
1206	Chopped or sliced	1 cup	180	94	38	2	1	0.1	0.1	0.2
1207	Slice, medium, ¼" thick	1 slice	20	94	4	Tr	Tr	Tr	Tr	Tr
	Whole									
1208	Cherry	1 cherry	17	94	4	Tr	Tr	Tr	Tr	Tr
1209	Medium, 2⅗" dia	1 tomato	123	94	26	1	Tr	0.1	0.1	0.2
1210	Canned, solids and liquid	1 cup	240	94	46	2	Tr	Tr	Tr	0.1
	Sun dried									
1211	Plain	1 piece	2	15	5	Tr	Tr	Tr	Tr	Tr
1212	Packed in oil, drained	1 piece	3	54	6	Tr	Tr	0.1	0.3	0.1
1213	Tomato juice, canned, with salt added	1 cup	243	94	41	2	Tr	Tr	Tr	0.1
	Tomato products, canned									
1214	Paste	1 cup	262	74	215	10	1	0.2	0.2	0.6
1215	Puree	1 cup	250	87	100	4	Tr	0.1	0.1	0.2
1216	Sauce	1 cup	245	89	74	3	Tr	0.1	0.1	0.2
	Spaghetti/marinara/pasta sauce. See Soups, Sauces, and Gravies.									
1217	Stewed	1 cup	255	91	71	2	Tr	Tr	0.1	0.1
1218	Turnips, cooked, cubes	1 cup	156	94	33	1	Tr	Tr	Tr	0.1
	Turnip greens, cooked, drained									
1219	From raw (leaves and stems)	1 cup	144	93	29	2	Tr	0.1	Tr	0.1
1220	From frozen (chopped)	1 cup	164	90	49	5	1	0.2	Tr	0.3
1221	Vegetable juice cocktail, canned	1 cup	242	94	46	2	Tr	Tr	Tr	0.1
	Vegetables, mixed									
1222	Canned, drained	1 cup	163	87	77	4	Tr	0.1	Tr	0.2
1223	Frozen, cooked, drained	1 cup	182	83	107	5	Tr	0.1	Tr	0.1
1224	Waterchestnuts, canned, slices, solids and liquids	1 cup	140	86	70	1	Tr	Tr	Tr	Tr

Miscellaneous Items

Food No.	Food Description	Measure of edible portion	Weight (g)	Water (%)	Calories (kcal)	Protein (g)	Total fat (g)	Saturated (g)	Monounsaturated (g)	Polyunsaturated (g)
1225	Bacon bits, meatless	1 tbsp	7	8	31	2	2	0.3	0.4	0.9
	Baking powders for home use									
	Double acting									
1226	Sodium aluminum sulfate	1 tsp	5	5	2	0	0	0.0	0.0	0.0
1227	Straight phosphate	1 tsp	5	4	2	Tr	0	0.0	0.0	0.0
1228	Low sodium	1 tsp	5	6	5	Tr	Tr	Tr	Tr	Tr
1229	Baking soda	1 tsp	5	Tr	0	0	0	0.0	0.0	0.0
1230	Beef jerky	1 large piece	20	23	81	7	5	2.1	2.2	0.2
1231	Catsup	1 cup	240	67	250	4	1	0.1	0.1	0.4
1232		1 tbsp	15	67	16	Tr	Tr	Tr	Tr	Tr
1233		1 packet	6	67	6	Tr	Tr	Tr	Tr	Tr
1234	Celery seed	1 tsp	2	6	8	Tr	1	Tr	0.3	0.1
1235	Chili powder	1 tsp	3	8	8	Tr	Tr	0.1	0.1	0.2
	Chocolate, unsweetened, baking									
1236	Solid	1 square	28	1	148	3	16	9.2	5.2	0.5
1237	Liquid	1 oz	28	1	134	3	14	7.2	2.6	3.0

*For product with no salt added: If salt added, consult the nutrition label for sodium value.

Miscellaneous Items (continued)

Food No.	Food Description	Measure of edible portion	Weight (g)	Water (%)	Calories (kcal)	Protein (g)	Total fat (g)	Fatty acids: Saturated (g)	Fatty acids: Monounsaturated (g)	Fatty acids: Polyunsaturated (g)
1238	Cinnamon	1 tsp	2	10	6	Tr	Tr	Tr	Tr	Tr
1239	Cocoa powder, unsweetened	1 cup	86	3	197	17	12	6.9	3.9	0.4
1240		1 tbsp	5	3	12	1	1	0.4	0.2	Tr
1241	Cream of tartar	1 tsp	3	2	8	0	0	0.0	0.0	0.0
1242	Curry powder	1 tsp	2	10	7	Tr	Tr	Tr	0.1	0.1
1243	Garlic powder	1 tsp	3	6	9	Tr	Tr	Tr	Tr	Tr
1244	Horseradish, prepared	1 tsp	5	85	2	Tr	Tr	Tr	Tr	Tr
1245	Mustard, prepared, yellow	1 tsp or 1 packet	5	82	3	Tr	Tr	Tr	0.1	Tr
	Olives, canned									
1246	Pickled, green	5 medium	17	78	20	Tr	2	0.3	1.6	0.2
1247	Ripe, black	5 large	22	80	25	Tr	2	0.3	1.7	0.2
1248	Onion powder	1 tsp	2	5	7	Tr	Tr	Tr	Tr	Tr
1249	Oregano, ground	1 tsp	2	7	5	Tr	Tr	Tr	Tr	0.1
1250	Paprika	1 tsp	2	10	6	Tr	Tr	Tr	Tr	0.2
1251	Parsley, dried	1 tbsp	1	9	4	Tr	Tr	Tr	Tr	Tr
1252	Pepper, black	1 tsp	2	11	5	Tr	Tr	Tr	Tr	Tr
	Pickles, cucumber									
1253	Dill, whole, medium (3¾" long)	1 pickle	65	92	12	Tr	Tr	Tr	Tr	0.1
1254	Fresh (bread and butter pickles), slices 1½" dia, ¼" thick	3 slices	24	79	18	Tr	Tr	Tr	Tr	Tr
1255	Pickle relish, sweet	1 tbsp	15	62	20	Tr	Tr	Tr	Tr	Tr
1256	Pork skins/rinds, plain	1 oz	28	2	155	17	9	3.2	4.2	1.0
	Potato chips									
	Regular									
	Plain									
1257	Salted	1 oz	28	2	152	2	10	3.1	2.8	3.5
1258	Unsalted	1 oz	28	2	152	2	10	3.1	2.8	3.5
1259	Barbecue flavor	1 oz	28	2	139	2	9	2.3	1.9	4.6
1260	Sour cream and onion flavor	1 oz	28	2	151	2	10	2.5	1.7	4.9
1261	Reduced fat	1 oz	28	1	134	2	6	1.2	1.4	3.1
1262	Fat free, made with olestra	1 oz	28	2	75	2	Tr	Tr	0.1	0.1
	Made from dried potatoes									
1263	Plain	1 oz	28	1	158	2	11	2.7	2.1	5.7
1264	Sour cream and onion flavor	1 oz	28	2	155	2	10	2.7	2.0	5.3
1265	Reduced fat	1 oz	28	1	142	2	7	1.5	1.7	3.8
1266	Salt	1 tsp	6	Tr	0	0	0	0.0	0.0	0.0
	Trail mix									
1267	Regular, with raisins, chocolate chips, salted nuts and seeds	1 cup	146	7	707	21	47	8.9	19.8	16.5
1268	Tropical	1 cup	140	9	570	9	24	11.9	3.5	7.2
1269	Vanilla extract	1 tsp	4	53	12	Tr	Tr	Tr	Tr	Tr
	Vinegar									
1270	Cider	1 tbsp	15	94	2	0	0	0.0	0.0	0.0
1271	Distilled	1 tbsp	17	95	2	0	0	0.0	0.0	0.0
	Yeast, baker's									
1272	Dry, active	1 pkg	7	8	21	3	Tr	Tr	0.2	Tr
1273		1 tsp	4	8	12	2	Tr	Tr	0.1	Tr
1274	Compressed	1 cake	17	69	18	1	Tr	Tr	0.2	Tr

Bibliography

ACSM's Guidelines for Exercise Testing and Prescription, 5th Edition, American College of Sports Medicine, Lippincott Williams & Wilkins, Hagerstown, MD 1995.

Fletcher, et. al., "Exercise Standards for Testing and Training," Circulation. 2001; 104:1694. American Heart Association, Inc.

U.S. Department of Agriculture, Agricultural Research Service. 2002. USDA Nutrient Database for Standard Reference, Release 15. Nutrient Data Laboratory Home Page, http://www.nal.usda.gov/fnic/foodcomp

About the author ...

I must first confess that I am not really a physics teacher. At least that's not what I started as ...

I graduated in Electrical Engineering from the University of Illinois – Urbana. While in school I worked in the co-op program and spent every other semester working at Hughes Aircraft in the missile development division. It was in college that I started bicycle racing. After graduation I took a job as an engineer at Motorola in the cellular subscriber division. I loved engineering and I enjoyed my job.

As I began to receive wider recognition as a bicycle racer, I accepted an offer to race full time. I raced all over the country, was selected to train at the Olympic Training Center, won 5 state titles, was twice named Illinois Rider of the Year, and rode in the 1992 Olympic Trials.

It was during the off-season one year that a physics teacher at a local high school quit – just didn't show up for work one day. A friend called and asked if I could just fill in until they could find a "real" teacher. The thought of teaching had never occurred to me and I had no experience, but I agreed. For 10 weeks I taught physics. It was by far the most demanding and challenging job I ever held. I was forced to draw on all my resources to teach in a way that was meaningful and valuable to the students. I drew on my own experiences in high school, college, many different engineering areas, and even my experiences in bike racing.

I loved engineering, but I felt a *calling* to be a teacher and that put teaching on a different level. After retiring from cycling I completed a Master's in education from Roosevelt University on Chicago and embarked on my teaching career.

This book is an extension of my passion for teaching. I hope you got something out of it. Not only in terms of weight loss, but also in terms of a little understanding of basic physics.

www.ingramcontent.com/pod-product-compliance
Lightning Source LLC
LaVergne TN
LVHW082353200926
848481LV00012B/3551
9780615148588